Applied Scientific Inquiry in the Health Professions: An Epistemological Orientation

Anne Cronin Mosey, PhD, OTR, FAOTA

Professor of Occupational Therapy
New York University

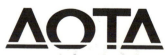

The American Occupational Therapy Association
Rockville, Maryland

"This publication is designed to provide accurate and authoritative information in regard to the subject matter covered. It is sold or distributed with the understanding that the publisher is not engaged in rendering legal, accounting, or other professional service. If legal advice or other expert assistance is required, the services of a competent professional person should be sought."

— From the Declaration of Principles jointly adopted by the American Bar Association and a Committee of Publishers and Associations.

It is the objective of the American Occupational Therapy Association to be a forum for free expression and interchange of ideas. The opinions and positions expressed by the contributors to this work are their own and not necessarily those of either the editors or the American Occupational Therapy Association.

Printed in the United States of America

Director of Publications: Anne M. Rosenstein
Design: Robert Sacheli
Editor: John Hutchins   **173395**

ISBN 0-910317-74-7

To My Father
Carlton R. Cronin
1910–1989

Acknowledgments

Many people influenced the preparation of this manuscript; some from long ago, some who surround me now. Each gave in their own way. But, in particular, I would like to acknowledge the help of:

Those who insisted I join the 20th Century before it is over and buy a computer,

The occupational and physical therapy students who raised and struggled with many of the questions addressed in the text,

Charles Paul Mosey, the family philosopher, and

Jim Hinojosa who kept the final watch.

To all of them a particular thank-you for the assistance, for making the process a learning experience, and for the many times when the doing was fun.

Preface

This text originated out of two questions: What is the nature of knowledge in the health professions—its origin, organization, and use? What is the appropriate form and focus of scientific inquiry in the health professions?

After I had reviewed the literature it became apparent that there were many points of view regarding the nature of knowledge and scientific inquiry. On closer reading, it was evident that these disparate views went far beyond semantics. Rather, there were fundamental differences in perspective grounded in diverse beliefs about professions, disciplines, knowledge, and science. The problem was not semantics; it was philosophical.

This text attempts to address the original questions by examining various philosophical—or, more correctly, epistemological—orientations, and then by discussing one orientation in depth. As part of the discussion of that orientation, the neopositivistic, a fairly detailed description of what is known about applied scientific inquiry is presented.

The text is designed to give entry-level professional students a way of looking at the knowledge they are in the process of mastering—its characteristics, how it fits together, where it comes from, and how it is used in daily practice. The text is also designed for postprofessional students and informed practitioners to facilitate study and discussion of the epistemology of practice, to assist in understanding applied scientific inquiry, and to use as a guide for doing applied inquiry. On a larger scale, it is hoped that the text will lead to a greater interest in the epistemology of practice and an appreciation of applied scientific inquiry. It is hoped these areas come to be examined more fully and argued more actively.

The text has been written for students and practitioners of all the health professions. It is not profession-specific because the issues addressed are common to all. However, my background as an occupational therapist is bound to have influenced some of my perceptions in ways in which I am unaware.

Some of the special concerns of occupational therapists, however, are addressed directly, particularly regarding the profession's sets of guidelines for practice, its frames of reference. In addition, a brief outline of occupational therapy's fundamental body of knowledge is presented in the Appendices.

Finally, despite what might be an abundance of new terms and definitions for the reader as well as some dense places in the text, I hope you enjoy.

Anne Cronin Mosey
August 1991

Table of Contents

Refining and Assessing the Adequacy of Sets of Guidelines

Some Observations on Sets of Guidelines for Practice

Developing Frames of Reference

Other Types of Sets of Guidelines for Practice

Section V—Postprofessional Education

Appendices: A Brief Outline of Occupational Therapy's Fundamental Body of Knowledge

Section I:
Introduction

The first two Chapters of this text provide a background for understanding applied scientific inquiry in the health professions. Applied scientific inquiry is defined and placed in an historical and contemporary context in Chapter 1. An area of investigation, epistemology of practice, is introduced as a philosophical framework for considering how knowledge is developed and used by practitioners. Four epistemological orientations that have been operant in the health professions are outlined in Chapter 2.

1. *From Practical to Applied Scientific Knowledge*

I n the past several years, health professions have become increasingly concerned about, and involved in, scientific inquiry. In so doing, many professions have raised questions about the nature and adequacy of their bodies of knowledge, the relationship between theory and practice, and the appropriate focus of scientific inquiry. Such questions belong in the realm of philosophy or, more specifically, *epistemology*—the investigation of the origin, nature, forms of inquiry, organization, beliefs associated with, and limits of human knowledge (Mitcham & Mackey, 1983; Wulff, Pedersen, & Rosenberg, 1986).

Philosophers have been concerned with epistemology for over 2,000 years. However, for the last 400 years or so, some philosophers have focused in particular on the epistemology of basic science and the process of basic science, as well as its end product—theory. There, for the most part, the study of the epistemology of science has stopped, as if there were nothing more. Philosophers have not studied the use of theoretical knowledge (Habermas, 1973). They have not investigated the way in which theoretical knowledge and the methods of science are employed to meet practical needs. As Bunge (1983) states, "the application of theory to practical goals poses considerable and largely neglected philosophical problems" (p. 62).

What has not developed, then, as an area of study is an epistemology of applied scientific inquiry. For now, *applied scientific inquiry* may be defined simply as a form of investigation that uses the methods of science and either theoretical information or research designs for the purpose of arriving at immediate practical ends. There are two distinct types of applied scientific inquiry that are sometimes confused: applied Type I and applied Type II.

Applied Type I scientific inquiry is the use of the methods of science and of theoretical information to formulate some sort of guidelines for action. In relation to health professions, these guidelines are referred to as *sets of guidelines for practice*—that is, integrated assemblages of information, extrapolated from theories and empirical data, that provide direction for identifying and resolving clinical problems with clients.

Applied Type II scientific inquiry is the use of the methods of science and research designs to answer specific practical questions. Typically, these are questions related to quantity, quality, value, safety, or effectiveness. Applied Type II scientific inquiry has two major foci. One, common in health professions, is refining and assessing the adequacy of sets of guidelines for practice. "Adequacy" refers to such matters as the reliability and validity of problem identification and the safety, effectiveness, efficiency, and acceptability to clients of the means employed for problem resolution.

The other focus of applied Type II scientific inquiry is addressing practical, topical questions about people, objects, and events, exemplified in the fields of epidemiology, demography, and consumer research. In the health professions, applied Type II inquiry is frequently employed to answer topical questions about the clients, educational activities, and the characteristics and opinions of members of their profession.

Applied scientific inquiry in the health professions is perhaps best understood by placing it in the broader context of epistemology of practice. The term *epistemology of practice* has been used by Schon (1983) in discussing Schein's (1972) work regarding levels of knowledge in science-based professions and in presenting his own ideas about the use of theoretical information (or the lack thereof) in professions. Schon did not define epistemology of practice, and, to the best of my knowledge, the term has not been used by others.

Thus, epistemology of practice is defined here as

investigation of the origin, nature, forms of inquiry, and organization of knowledge in the science-based professions and the use of such knowledge in practice. It also includes study of how professions describe their ideology and its relationship to scientific knowledge. Epistemology of practice, as defined here, is not concerned with parapractice knowledge—that is, knowledge related to administration and consultation, for example.

This text is about applied scientific inquiry and the epistemology of practice in health professions. *Health professions* are, first and foremost, professions—occupational groups recognized by society as having expertise in assisting people in resolving specified practical problems. Professions are responsible for developing the applied body of knowledge upon which their practice is based and for using that knowledge in such a way as to directly benefit society.

Second, health professions are science-based. As such, they are responsible for assisting people through the use of applied knowledge that is derived from the most valid theoretical information currently available (M. S. Larsen, 1977). Professions like law and the clergy are not considered to be science-based, for example, because their supporting bodies of knowledge are founded on information outside of the realm of science (Hughes, 1973). Third, health professions, as the name implies, are concerned with problems related to health and, by extension, illness, disability, and lack of health. They may be distinguished from other science-based professions, such as education and engineering, that assist individuals with practical problems that are typically not directly related to health. Of course, the purposes of professions frequently overlap.

Lack of attention to the epistemology of practice on the part of practitioners is probably due to several factors: preoccupation with assisting clients, no pressing feeling of urgency to examine the subject, and hesitancy to enter a new area of study. More generally, neglect of the epistemology of practice and, by extension, the epistemology of applied scientific inquiry by both practitioners and philosophers seems to be associated with a cluster of interrelated negative attitudes. These attitudes are grounded in the distinction between *praxis* and *theoria* made by ancient Greek philosophers. They have been reinforced by the evolution of divergent roles for disciplines and professions regarding the development and use of scientific knowledge.

Praxis and Theoria

Practical knowledge is the signature of our immediate ancestors and parents written in their tools, their hearths, their amulets and beads. We identify them as like us because of their *praxis*—their use of practical knowledge. Our ancestors' and parents' knowledge was that of making, inventing, controlling, and providing care for each other. Such knowledge was created and advanced through *practical inquiry*—observation, reasoning, trial and error, and taking advantage of fortuitous happenings. Praxis was used to fulfill everyday needs and desires. In conjunction with knowledge about the supernatural, praxis served and sustained humankind for thousands of years, up until the time of the Greeks.[1]

Around 600 BC, a new type of knowledge was sought. Initiated by the Ionians, the knowledge was neither practical nor of a supernatural nature; rather, it was concerned with formulating general principles—*theoria*—to explain the nature and organization of the universe. Methods of inquiry were refined and used: observation, speculation, and reasoning. Investigation was motivated only by the wish to know and understand, not for any practical purpose. Philosophy began.

The development of practical knowledge continued, of course, but separate from philosophical knowledge. The praxis of craftsmen, physicians, and artisans was quite different than the theoria of philosophers. Praxis was concerned with the solution of practical problems, theoria with the universe. Greek philosophers recognized the necessity of praxis but viewed it as far inferior to theoria. Theoria was knowledge writ large, praxis was... just praxis. It is not known how craftsmen and artisans viewed theoria. One could speculate that perhaps they thought theoria was... just theoria. There was little recognized interrelationship

---

[1] The following historical overview is based on the work of Grove (1989), Hellemans and Bunch (1988), Kneller (1978), Rosenberg and Birdzell (1990), Tempkin (1977), Van Melsen (1961), and Wulff, Pedersen, and Rosenberg (1986).

Applied Scientific Inquiry in the Health Professions

or interaction between theoria and praxis; each developed separately and in its own way. The one exception seems to be a school of Greek physicians who, in part, used some ideas from the philosophy of their time. They loosely equated the four elements—air, fire, earth, and water—with four bodily humors—blood, yellow bile, black bile, and phlegm (Ackerknecht, 1968).

It was not until about the middle of the 16th century, through the work of Copernicus, Galileo, Bacon, and many others, that modern science begin to emerge from philosophy. Reliance on the authority of past and present philosophers was viewed as detrimental to the advancement of knowledge. Moreover, it was felt that at least some knowledge was best acquired through direct observation and the verification of observation through experimentation. Reasoning remained important, but reliance on reasoning or speculation alone was suspect.

This new pursuit, natural philosophy, was not concerned with the universe in its entirety but only with the physical world, that which could be directly observed and measured. The insubstantial, the essence of reality, the nature of knowledge, esthetics, and moral behavior remained within the domain of philosophy. It took science nearly 400 years to develop into its modern form separate from philosophy. The final step, at least symbolically, took place toward the end of the 19th century when natural philosophers, at the urging of Whewell, began to refer to themselves as "scientists" (Hellemans & Bunch, 1988).

Basic scientists, using agreed-upon methods of inquiry and research designs, saw their task as developing general principles to explain the nature of the physical universe. This new kind of knowledge came to be known as *theory*, a derivative of theoria. However, the theory of science is of quite a different order and is more strictly structured than the theoria of philosophy. Scientific theory is an abstract description of a circumscribed set of physical phenomena that delineates the characteristics of the phenomena and their relationship to each other. Examples of scientific theories are anatomy, thermodynamics, and operant conditioning. The magnitude of the phenomena addressed by a theory may be comparatively small, as in biomechanics, or much larger, as in the general theory of relativity. The search for an all encompassing scientific theory, which is similar to some philosophers' quests for a general theoria, remains viable in at least some of the scientific disciplines.

As basic science developed, so too did practical knowledge continue to develop, accumulate, and become more refined. The inquiries of the practitioner and the basic scientist were in many ways similar. Both involved observation, experimentation (in the form of trial and error), reasoning, and the use of fortuitous happenings. The major difference between practical inquiry and basic scientific inquiry was that practitioners were not concerned with identifying general principles. Rather, their goal was finding a practical solution to whatever problem was at hand. Principles that explain the physical universe were not of concern to the practitioner.

With some exceptions, it was not until the middle of the 19th century that what are now considered to be science-based professions began to question the use of practical inquiry alone as a means of enhancing practice. Increasingly, they became aware of the possibility of using knowledge generated through basic scientific inquiry and of using this theoretical information as the foundation for dealing with practical problems. They also began to recognize the usefulness of more strict adherence to the methods of science and the advantage of various research designs. This was the beginning of applied scientific inquiry.

It has taken some time for the goals and processes of applied scientific inquiry to emerge and be recognized. This text is one example in a long line of efforts to articulate the nature of applied scientific inquiry. Change from practical inquiry to applied scientific inquiry was gradual, first affecting chemical industries and military engineering, then, at the start of the 20th century, medicine, education, and, by the 1940s, most other forms of engineering and the health professions. The relationship that evolved between basic science (scientific disciplines) and applied science (science-based professions) is discussed in the next section.

Philosophy and basic science are now seen as fairly distinct enterprises, but a strong bond remains between them. Some philosophers have selected basic science as their area of study. Philosophy of science is an active field of inquiry concerned with investigating many facets of basic science: its fundamental beliefs, its ethical issues, the relationship between basic science and society, basic science as a human activity, and the epistemology of basic science.

Philosophers have also contributed to the understanding of professions (Mitcham & Mackey, 1983). They have explored the assumptions, beliefs, and values professions espouse and bring to practice as well as the relationship between practice and society. In conjunction with such study, they have also considered the ethics of practice, often assisting professions in developing standards of ethical practice.

What philosophers have not explored is the epistemology of practice. One reason for this has been suggested. In summary, Greek philosophers and those who followed did not see praxis, practical knowledge, as knowledge. If it was knowledge, it was at such a low level that it did not deserve consideration. To some extent, the theoria of philosophers evolved into scientific theory; praxis became theoretically based, applied knowledge. Yet the attitudes of most of today's philosophers of science toward applied knowledge remain similar to the ancient attitude toward praxis: it is not worthy of study.

Disciplines and Professions

The second factor that has contributed to the neglect of the epistemologies of practice and applied scientific inquiry is the division of labor that has evolved between the scientific disciplines and the science-based professions. Each has a different role in the development and use of basic scientific knowledge.[2]

In general, *disciplines* are occupational groups recognized by society as having expertise in scholarly inquiry directed toward specified categories of phenomena. Each discipline is responsible for advancing knowledge about phenomena within its sphere of study.

---

[2] Discussion of these divergent roles is based on the work of Altmaier and Meyer (1985), Dingwall (1982), Fox (1986), Goodlad (1984), Lieb (1986), McGlothlin (1964), J. C. Rogers (1983), and Snelbecker (1974).

More specifically, scientific disciplines are responsible for inquiry directed toward defined categories of physical phenomena for the purpose of developing valid theories that allow for accurate prediction about the phenomena addressed. Some theoretical information is free-floating, however—that is, it is not yet organized into the formal structure of a theory—and can be referred to as *empirical data*. (The term, "theoretical information," when used in the text, refers to both theories and empirical data.) Examples of scientific disciplines are physics, chemistry, and biology. Disciplines such as theology, history, and English literature are differentiated from the scientific disciplines since their scholarly inquiry is directed toward goals other than the development of scientific theories. Science-based professions were previously defined (see page 5).

The complex relationship between scientific disciplines (disciplines), science-based professions (professions), and society is presented in Figure 1. A more complete description appears in Chapter 9.

Through the use of basic scientific inquiry, disciplines formulate, refine, and test theoretical information—and there it ends. There is no immediate link between theoretical information and society. (Thus, no line connects these two entities in Figure 1.) The absence of an immediate link is due to one of the primary characteristics of theoretical information: it cannot be directly applied (Glaser, 1976; Hilgard & Bower, 1974). Theoretical information is descriptive only and, in and of itself, offers no suggestion for application. For example, one cannot directly apply human anatomy or Freud's theory of psychosexual development. In order to be used, theoretical information must be transformed into sets of guidelines for practice. Formulating valid theory is the only responsibility of disciplines. Application is not expected from disciplines, nor is it within their domain.

Conversely, professions are concerned with application of theoretical information. Using applied Type I scientific inquiry, professions select potentially suitable theories and empirical data from the fund of basic knowledge available from the disciplines. (This is illustrated in Figure 1 by the descending line from theoretical information to professions.) Professions then

Figure 1. A schematic representation of the relationship between the basic scientific inquiry of disciplines, the applied scientific inquiry of professions, and assisting society with practical problems.

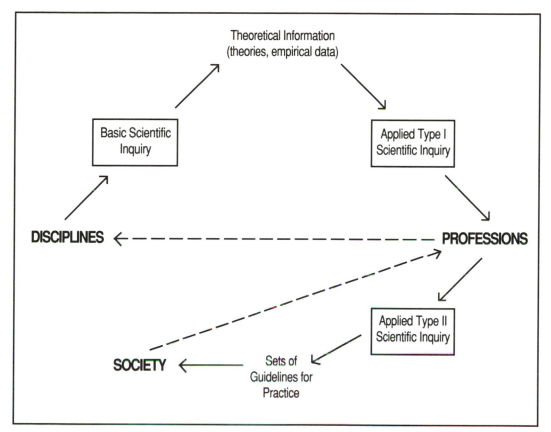

extrapolate from this theoretical information and, through deductive and inductive reasoning, develop tentative sets of guidelines for practice. For example, medicine draws on theoretical information from physiology and anatomy to use as the foundation for the diagnosis and treatment of appendicitis.

Subsequently, through the use of applied Type II inquiry, sets of guidelines for practice are refined, and their adequacy is assessed. They are used to assist society in satisfying its various needs. (This is illustrated by the unbroken line from profession to society in Figure 1.) Without the applied scientific inquiry of professions, the theoretical information of disciplines would not be used, nor would society receive the benefits of theoretical knowledge generated through basic scientific inquiry.

Communication between society, professions, and

disciplines is represented by the broken lines in Figure 1. Society seeks assistance from professions to meet its various identified needs (the ascending line from society to professions). When no suitable theoretical information is available for formulating adequate sets of guidelines for practice, professions turn to appropriate disciplines for development of such information (illustrated by the directional, broken line between professions and disciplines).

The relationships between disciplines and professions—between basic and applied scientific inquiry—will be looked at more thoroughly later; however, several general points should be made here. First, the goals and end products of disciplines and professions are different. The work of disciplines and professions may be interactive, but they are not the same. Second, with some notable exceptions, the scientific inquiry of disciplines and of professions is somewhat distant in time and place. Theoretical information may be developed long before it is used; basic scientific inquiry typically takes place in a laboratory setting whereas applied scientific inquiry tends to occur more in the immediacy of a practical problem—in a clinic, for example. Finally, applied scientific inquiry is a relatively new activity. The interaction between disciplines and professions described here has only been happening for a fairly short period of time.

Although the relationship between disciplines and professions is usually one of respect and cooperation, there is sometimes a more unpleasant side. Almost since the beginning of modern science, people within the scientific disciplines have emphasized the practical benefits to be gained from basic scientific inquiry—especially when seeking financial support for some project. However, there is little evidence of any dedication to the idea, among the scientific disciplines, that the purpose of basic scientific inquiry is to enhance the daily life of humankind. As Campbell (1980) comments, "there is surely no more damning word in the lexicon of the true disciplinarian than 'applied'" (p. 174).

Many in the scientific disciplines do not view applied scientific inquiry as belonging in the realm of science (Singleton, Straits, Straits, & McAllister, 1988). Others tentatively accept applied scientific inquiry as a part of science, but see those who engage in such inquiry as having a lesser calling and as being unable to attain the intellectual sophistication required to engage in basic scientific inquiry (Mitcham & Mackey, 1983; Skolimowski, 1983). Applied scientists, above all, are tainted with praxis. Since the majority of philosophers of science received their graduate education in one of the scientific disciplines and worked within that discipline prior to turning their attention to philosophy, their neglect of and, at times, rejection of applied scientific inquiry may be the result of attitudes acquired early in their careers.

Basic scientists and philosophers of basic science have been frequent champions of the superiority of basic scientific inquiry over applied scientific inquiry. Society, on the whole, has accepted this idea and the negative attitudes associated with it. Some health practitioners may also be unwitting carriers of these prejudicial attitudes—attitudes that this text seeks to dispel.

Prior to proceeding, the similarities between epistemology of practice and epistemology of technology, also an emerging area of study, should be noted (Ihde, 1983; Kneller, 1978; Mitcham & Mackey, 1983; Phillips, 1987; Van Melsen, 1961; Williams, 1974a). These similarities are particularly apparent in the area of applied scientific inquiry, a form of investigation common to both. The end products of applied Type I scientific inquiry in technological professions are *sets of technological guidelines*—integrated assemblages of information, extrapolated from theories and/or empirical data, that provide direction for fabricating technological products. Thus, the end products of applied Type I scientific inquiry can be seen as *sets of guidelines for action*, with two major sub-divisions:

1. Sets of guidelines for practice
2. Sets of technological guidelines

Applied Type II inquiry is also employed extensively in technological professions to refine and assess the adequacy of sets of technological guidelines and products as well as to address topical questions.

Work done in the area of epistemology of technology is used in the text to explore and elucidate the epistemologies of practice and applied scientific inquiry. Although the epistemologies of applied scientific inquiry and practice are the primary focus of this text, the place of technology in practice is briefly described in Chapter 4.

About this Book

As outlined in the last two sections, historical and contemporary attitudes toward practice and applied scientific inquiry have impeded study of the knowledge formulated by, and used in, health professions. Nevertheless, the examination of such knowledge now has a name: the epistemology of practice. Naming something is not the same as understanding it, but it is an initial step in that direction.

As a framework for understanding applied scientific inquiry, this book begins with an investigation of the epistemology of practice. A survey of the health professions' literature reveals a number of different ideas about the nature of knowledge fundamental to practice. From these ideas, four relatively discrete epistemological orientations have been identified. Three of these—traditional, disciplinal, and phenomenological—will be briefly reviewed. The fourth, neopositivistic, will be considered in depth.

The neopositivistic orientation is examined in detail for three reasons. First, it seems to be the current orientation, in whole or in part, of the majority of the health professions, whether or not it is consciously recognized by these professions as the predominant orientation. It should be recognized, however, that neopositivism is not the professed epistemological orientation of some health professions. It is also strongly opposed by some health professionals. Second, the neopositivistic orientation, more than any of the others, seems to provide an orderly and systematic description of the knowledge fundamental to practice. Third, and most importantly, the neopositivistic orientation provides the foundation for understanding and engaging in applied scientific inquiry. Applied scientific inquiry is an inherent part of the neopositivistic orientation, supporting and giving meaning to its use by the health professions. This is not the case with the other three epistemological orientations.

The neopositivistic epistemological orientation to practice is founded on three interrelated assumptions:

1. Practice in the health professions is based on

diverse theoretical information drawn from a variety of disciplines.

2. Scientific theories and empirical data cannot be directly applied.

3. Applied scientific inquiry is the process whereby theoretical information is transformed in such a way that it can be used as the foundation for practice.

After the discussion of the neopositivistic orientation, this book turns to applied scientific inquiry. The nature of applied scientific inquiry is described, and the process of how one goes about engaging in applied scientific inquiry is explained. Emphasis is placed on that aspect of applied scientific inquiry concerned with developing, refining, and assessing the adequacy of theoretically based sets of guidelines for practice. Although this portion of the text is primarily didactic and intended for instruction, it is also exploratory because there is much that is not known about applied scientific inquiry.

Applied scientific inquiry cannot be understood or engaged in with any skill without knowledge of basic scientific inquiry. Therefore, basic inquiry is discussed from the perspective of applied inquiry to provide an understanding of:

1. Science in general and the methods of science.

2. The nature of theoretical information.

3. Those aspects of theoretical information that must be taken into consideration when engaging in applied Type I scientific inquiry.

In conclusion, the epistemologies of practice and applied scientific inquiry are areas of study that have received little attention. The questions addressed in this text may not be the right questions. If some of the right questions are being addressed, fruitful answers may not be within these pages. And that is as it should be, for the purpose of this text is to take a few steps in the initial phase of a journey. There are mostly blank spaces on the map; exploration of the terrain has just begun. As Scott and Shore (1979) point out, how science influences the conduct of practical activities is an extremely complex problem.

2. Four Epistemological Orientations to Practice

T he four epistemological orientations to practice described here are distilled from the literature of various health professions and the literature about allied health professions. They are outlined in a pure form and described as if they actually existed as separate entities. In reality, overlap among the orientations exists as they are reflected in any given health profession. Some professions have two fairly distinct epistemological orientations; others seem to be in the process of changing from one orientation to another.

The descriptions here have been synthesized to emphasize the special characteristics of each epistemological orientation. Discussion is structured around the areas of study identified in the definition of epistemology of practice: origin, nature, ideology, form of inquiry, organization, and use.

Origin refers to what is considered to be the source of knowledge in a profession, that from which it arises or is derived. It concerns beliefs about what is the proper knowledge of a profession.

Nature refers to the characteristics of the knowledge most directly used in practice. It concerns the form of that knowledge as well as its constituent parts and their properties. An example of "knowledge most directly used" is the diagnostic categories of medicine.

Ideology refers to the values and beliefs of a profession regarding the individual, the environment, the relationship between the individual and the environment, and the purpose and goals of the profession.

The role of ideology varies from one epistemological orientation to another; it may be considered very important—or of little concern. Of particular interest here will be the relationship between ideology and scientific knowledge.

Form of inquiry refers to what a profession inquires about, the methods it uses, and how it develops, refines, and evaluates knowledge. It concerns the process of how new knowledge is added and how ineffectual knowledge is deleted from a profession's body of knowledge.

Organization refers to the way in which a profession's body of knowledge is ordered as a whole. It concerns the parts of that whole, the way the parts are structured in relationship to each other, and their interdependence.

Use refers to how knowledge is selected and applied in the immediacy of the situation of practice. It refers to how information guides the process of problem identification and resolution.

It should be noted that some areas of study are more suitable for describing one epistemological orientation than others. This will become apparent in the discussion of each of the orientations. While the four orientations will not be compared in a critical manner, a few comments will be offered regarding the advantages and disadvantages of each. Figure 2, located at the end of the chapter (page 42), provides an overview of the four orientations.

The Traditional Orientation

The traditional epistemological orientation to practice must actually be described in retrospect. There are no professions in which this orientation is currently dominant. It is presented here for three reasons:

1. It will give some perspective to the other three orientations, a way of looking at the present by momentarily looking at the past.
2. The traditional orientation, to some degree, remains operant and influential in many professions. Most professions continue to rely on some unexamined information, some folk knowledge from the past.
3. Practical inquiry, a part of this orientation, may be employed as a last resort when scientific inquiry fails to yield useful information.

All practitioners are influenced by the traditional orientation, but their awareness of this influence varies; they may be completely unaware or comfortably aware, or they may be slightly haunted by its influence.

The beginnings of most professions lie hidden in the mist of antiquity. Nevertheless, professions often study their history, finding traces of their present practices in the past, identifying historical figures who influenced the profession, and naming the modern founders. Somewhere in the history of a profession there is a discernible time when the profession begins to develop a coherent scientific foundation. Terms such as *theory*, *science*, and *research* begin to appear in the literature. This is the beginning of the scientific period of the profession. The prior, prescientific period is the time of a traditional epistemological orientation (Ackerknecht, 1968; Anderson & Bell, 1988; Downs, 1979; Flexner, 1910; Gurin & Williams, 1973; Horgan, 1988). Readers from professions other than medicine can perhaps best get a feel for this orientation by examining their professional journals from before the early 1950s.

Origin   In a traditional orientation, knowledge fundamental to practice was embedded in the past. It was transferred from one generation to the next with only small increments of change. Current practice was based on the practical wisdom of those who had gone before. Although some didactic instruction was provided, education by apprenticeship was considered the best way to ensure mastery of the profession's body of knowledge.

Nature   Knowledge consisted of *particular solutions* to specific problems. There was no range of solutions for a particular problem; instead, there was one particular solution. A system of conventional rules governed the ways things were done, and on the whole these rules were followed. The use of such particularized solutions is now sometimes pejoratively referred to as "the cookbook approach."

An example from occupational therapy may help to illustrate. In preparation for working in psychiatry, students were given a list of particular solutions for dealing with various symptoms such as depression, anger, anxiety, and so forth. For each symptom, specific activities were prescribed, and the appropriate behavior by the therapist was described. The list was memorized to be used in the clinic.

Ideology	Practitioners within a traditional orientation usually had little awareness of the values and belief systems underlying their profession. However, when the values were codified or articulated in some way, they were rarely questioned. Since these were the supposedly agreed-upon beliefs and values of the profession, there was no need for discussion or study.
Form of inquiry	When the knowledge of traditional professions did change, it did so at a very slow pace. Practical inquiry was used at times to find a different particular solution for a problem. Inquiry also sometimes involved, as Sloane nicely states, "analysis of the deeds successfully done" (Anderson & Bell, 1988, p. 9). Particular solutions, however, were not subject to rigorous assessment regarding their safety or effectiveness. Solutions believed to be effective were often not; some were even detrimental. Bloodletting is a classic example. There was little, if any, questioning of the effectiveness of a particular solution because, on the whole, there was no general spirit of inquiry. Indeed, inquiry was often discouraged. New particular solutions were suspect. Acceptance of change was grudging and controversial.
Organization	There was only one level of knowledge in the traditional orientation. The body of knowledge consisted of particular solutions. No fundamental body of knowledge served as the basis for developing particular solutions, nor guided how particular solutions were selected and used in practice.
Use	The use of knowledge in the traditional orientation is probably quite apparent from what has been described above. There was a one-to-one relationship between problem and solution. While a particular solution—for example, bed rest—may have been used to ameliorate several different problems, a given problem rarely had more than one recommended solution.
Comments	The major beneficiary of a profession with a traditional epistemological orientation is probably the student practitioner. Although apprenticeship training may have been lengthy, there were particular solutions to most problems. When no solution was available, nothing could be done. There were none of the unknowns and complexities that hold contemporary students to their desks late into the night.

The disadvantages of professions based on the traditional orientation are fairly obvious. Problem identification and resolution were primitive. Intervention was frequently not effective and was, at times, unsafe. Moreover, knowledge was slow to advance because a profession based on the authority of the past does not easily embrace innovative ideas. Finally, with no larger pool of knowledge to draw upon, traditional professions were without the "cognitive capital" of science (Merton, 1982).

The Disciplinal Orientation

The disciplinal epidemiological orientation to practice is named to reflect its major tenet: professions are responsible for developing, refining, and testing the validity of their theoretical body of knowledge. As such, they are "like disciplines." The division of labor between disciplines and professions, in which disciplines develop and professions use theoretical knowledge (outlined in Chapter 1), is not recognized or accepted. Professions with a disciplinal orientation try not to draw upon the bodies of knowledge of the various disciplines.[1]

A theoretical body of knowledge, central to the disciplinal orientation, tends to be organized into one of two formats, although these formats may overlap. One format is a single all-inclusive conceptual system, which may be referred to by many names: paradigm, meta-theory, unifying concepts, model, the theory of [the name of the profession], and comprehensive theory. In this text, the system will be called *comprehensive theory*—a highly abstract theory with rather loose boundaries that addresses a broad spectrum of phenomena through the use of fairly global, open-ended concepts (Merton, 1982; Mills, 1967). The comprehensive theory of a profession with a disciplinal orientation addresses all of the phenomena of concern to the profession and contains all of the theoretical information used by the profession.

---

[1] The following discussion is based on the ideas presented by Beckstrand (1986), Christiansen (1990), Dickoff and James (1968), Fitzpatrick and Whall (1983), Fleming, Johnson, Marina, Spergel, and Townson (1987), and Kielhofner (1983).

The other format for organizing theoretical knowledge in the disciplinal orientation is a collection of individual theories, each addressing a relatively circumscribed set of phenomena. These theories are formulated by the profession for its own purposes. The individual theories are far less global than comprehensive theories, describing only a limited range of phenomena within the broader category of phenomena of concern to the profession. Concepts are more narrow and specifically defined. This format will be referred to as *multiple theories*. Regardless of the format they use, proponents of this orientation believe that the theoretical body of knowledge of a profession is similar to the body of knowledge of a discipline.

Origin
The origin of the disciplinal orientation is described in two parts: (a) the genesis of the orientation itself and (b) the genesis of the two formats, a comprehensive theory and multiple-theories.

Genesis of the Orientation
The disciplinal orientation began to develop when health professions, beginning with medicine, recognized that basic scientific knowledge could make a significant contribution to the purpose and goals of their profession (see Chapter 1, page 7). Concomitant with this recognition was the acceptance of *rational empiricism*—the belief that basic scientific knowledge is best acquired through a combination of logical reasoning, observation, and procedures for verifying observations (Hellemans & Bunch, 1988; Wulff, Pedersen, & Rosenberg, 1986). Reason or observation alone were not considered to lead to sound scientific knowledge. With acceptance of these ideas, a profession moves from a traditional orientation to being science-based.

This transition has been shared by many professions. What distinguishes professions choosing the disciplinal orientation over the neopositivistic orientation are two additional founding ideas:

1. Theoretical information can be directly applied.
2. To be truly science-based, a profession must have a theoretical body of knowledge that it alone has formulated.

Genesis of Formats
The genesis of comprehensive theories varies as does the motivation for their development. At the risk of considerable simplification, three somewhat different sources are identified and illustrated through examples.

Applied Scientific Inquiry in the Health Professions

One source is perhaps best described as *ex post facto*. A comprehensive theory is formulated from seemingly disparate, accumulated scientific data that are brought together into one theoretical system. This theory comes to serve as the knowledge base of a profession. An example is the germ theory of disease (Hallemans & Bunch, 1988). This comprehensive theory was synthesized from the work of Pasteur, Laveran, and others who identified various organisms—bacteria, protozoa, fungi, and eventually viruses—as the causal factors in a variety of diseases. This theory began to be popularly used by medicine at the end of the 19th century. (It should be noted that medicine no longer has a disciplinal orientation; it is now neopositivistic.)

Another source of comprehensive theory comes from a profession's need to establish its identity. This is perhaps best illustrated by Dickoff and James (1968) in their description of the need for a comprehensive theory for nursing. A comprehensive theory "must go beyond describing, explaining and predicting phenomena—it must provide a conceptualization intended to guide the shaping of reality to a professional purpose" (p. 198). Such comprehensive theories tend to be *a priori* in that, on the whole, they are formulated prior to seeking data for their support. Examples include the theories of nursing developed by M. E. Rogers (1970) and King (1981). The model of human occupation, once viewed as a comprehensive theory for occupational therapy, is another example (Kielhofner, 1983).

The third source of comprehensive theory seems to be the need to fill some sort of a theoretical vacuum in a profession or in society. This is exemplified in psychoanalytic theory. Developed by Freud and his colleagues and intellectual heirs, psychoanalytic theory is an explanation of human behavior using the construct of the unconscious as an explanatory device. Psychoanalytic theory served as the comprehensive theory for psychiatry for nearly 50 years.

The genesis of the multiple-theories format in the disciplinal orientation is closely related to how a profession delimits its theoretical domain—that is, the "relatively circumscribed category of phenomena" it considered to be its own. How this domain is defined is not entirely clear, however. The areas of human function of concern to the profession, its beliefs about the goals and purposes of the profession, and the media or tools it has traditionally used all seem to be factors. At some point the profession identifies its domain of study, and theory development begins.

Nature In the disciplinal orientation, a profession's theoretical knowledge is seen as unique, not shared by any other profession or discipline. This is true regardless of whether a comprehensive theory or a multiple-theories format is espoused. Theoretical knowledge not within the comprehensive theory or multiple-theories is viewed as highly suspect. However, the use of such information in practice is tolerated only because it is seen as temporary; the use of "outside" information will diminish as the profession increases its own fund of theoretical knowledge.

In addition to what has been described, comprehensive theories often have one or more of the characteristics described below (Mosey, 1985):

Comprehensive theories are seen as monistic—that is, based on a first principle that is identified as the essence of reality. Monism is the belief that all processes, structures, concepts, and theories can be reduced to one governing principle (Marx & Cronan-Hillix, 1987). Two examples are "germs cause all diseases" and "the unconscious influences all behavior."

Holism—the position that entities should be studied and dealt with as whole units—is another characteristic attributed to some comprehensive theories. This is considered by some to be the opposite of reductionism—the position that, to some extent at least, entities are best understood through consideration of parts (Marx & Cronan-Hillix, 1987).

Comprehensive theories are often viewed as dominant, governing or determining all aspects of the profession. Ideas or activities perceived as incompatible with the comprehensive theory are seriously questioned. The theory is used as a filter to determine what ideas and activities will and will not be considered legitimate to the profession.

Theories in a multiple-theories format may have the typical characteristics of theories (see Chapter 8), or they may contain information usually not included in theories, such as information about application.

Where this additional information regarding application comes from and how it is derived is not clear; applied Type I inquiry is not part of the disciplinal orientation. Theories with this additional information are treated as theories, not some other, different type of conceptual system.

Ideology   When a profession has a comprehensive theory, no strong distinction is made between the beliefs of the profession and its comprehensive theory. The comprehensive theory is viewed as part of the ideology of the profession. No line is drawn so that one can easily say, "this is a philosophical statement" or "this is a theoretical statement." Ideology tends to be separate from theoretical information in professions with a multiple-theories format, however. It also seems to play a less dominant role than in professions with comprehensive theories. The place of ideology in such professions relative to organization of knowledge seems to be rather vague.

Form of Inquiry   Basic scientific inquiry is the primary form of investigation in the disciplinal orientation because one of the fundamental tenets of this epistemological orientation is the belief that theoretical knowledge can be directly used in practice. No intermediary step, information, conceptual system, or body of knowledge is required. Therefore, inquiry is directed toward developing, refining, and testing the validity of the comprehensive theory or collection of multiple theories.

Some professions with a disciplinal orientation do see a limited role for applied scientific inquiry, but only as secondary to basic inquiry. Although applied Type I inquiry is not recognized in the disciplinal professions, applied Type II inquiry is considered useful for developing evaluative tools and sometimes for assessing the effectiveness of intervention. At other times, the process of assessing the effectiveness of intervention tests the theory being used. Thus, investigation would entail the use of basic scientific inquiry.

Organization   There is usually only one level in the organization of knowledge in a disciplinal epistemological orientation to practice. The hierarchial structure of some comprehensive theories demarcates levels within the theory, but this does not indicate levels of knowledge because the comprehensive theory or multiple theories are treated as if they are the entirety of the profession's body of knowledge. More than one level of organization is implied in a multiple-theories format, but there does not seem to be any typical pattern of organization across professions.

Use How knowledge is actually used in a disciplinal orientation is not exactly clear. In other words, it is often not specified how the comprehensive theory/multiple theories relate to practice. This may or may not be recognized by the proponents of this orientation. For some, formulating a comprehensive theory is seen as a first step, to be followed by development of theories derived from the comprehensive theory. These theories, more limited in scope, are to be used as the basis for practice. Others take the position that it is not theories that will be derived from the comprehensive theory but some other type of conceptual system that, in turn, will be used as the basis for practice. This need for "some other type of conceptual system" is recognized but rarely defined. When it is defined, the conceptual system seems much like the "sets of guidelines for practice" of the neopositivistic orientation. Rarely, however, are conceptual systems for application actually derived from the comprehensive theory; the scholarly work of the profession usually remains focused on the comprehensive theory.

When the need to relate comprehensive theory to practice is not recognized by a profession, one of two approaches are taken. Some comprehensive theories include the concept of an "open system"—any entity that is influenced by the environment and in turn influences the environment (Bertalanffy, 1967). A continuous cycle is postulated in which the entity is changed as it interacts with the environment, and the environment is changed as the entity interacts with it. Therefore, practice is viewed as assisting the individual (an open system) through his or her interaction in a somewhat controlled or specially designed environment. However, the comprehensive theory rarely provides information about how the environment should be arranged and what behavior is to be encouraged.

The other approach is what Judith Larsen (1981) refers to as "conceptual utilization." In this situation, the comprehensive theory serves as a way of thinking about practice—it is not directly used but rather forms a context for action. Again, specific information regarding practice is not usually provided. When a profession has a multiple-theories format, with or without "information about application," these theories are directly applied. However, in most cases their application seems to be more accurately described as "conceptual utilization."

Regardless of the format of a profession's theoretical body of knowledge, information about practice in the disciplinal orientation tends to be provided through presentation of case studies.

Comments The primary advantage of a disciplinal orientation with a comprehensive theory format is the feeling of identity and unity that it gives to a profession. It provides a sense of direction; general goals seem to be clear with regard to the focus of intervention and scientific inquiry. However, because of the limitations just described regarding use, the profession's sense of security may be illusory.

Some of the characteristics of comprehensive theory—monism, inclusion of ideology, and dominance of the theory—may place the profession in a constricted position in which the theory becomes so central and requires such a degree of loyalty that creative, divergent, independent thinking is not encouraged or perhaps even tolerated. New ideas, new scientific data, and the changing needs of society may not be given sufficient attention (Mosey, 1985).

The intertwining of ideology and theoretical information, typical in comprehensive theory, makes it difficult to determine the difference between a statement of belief and a theoretical statement. What type of scholarly activity to pursue may not be apparent. Should one, for example, engage in philosophical inquiry or basic scientific inquiry?

There are two other problems related to basic scientific inquiry relative to a comprehensive theory. One is the highly abstract nature of such theories that makes them hard to test. It is difficult to formulate operational definitions for global, open-ended concepts. By the time concepts are reduced to the level of variables, the variables often bear little resemblance to the original concepts. This is exemplified by the difficulty in fomulating an operational definition for concepts such as "id" and "ego" from psychoanalytic theory. Thus, tested hypotheses may be so distant from the comprehensive theory that findings cannot, with any honesty, be used to verify the postulates from which the hypotheses are deduced. The other problem relative to basic scientific inquiry relates back to the issue of ideology. There is often such a strong feeling the comprehensive theory is "right," that findings not supportive of the theory are ignored or ascribed to faulty research design. Such a situation is not conducive to sound scientific inquiry.

Of the several problems related to a comprehensive theory format, the major difficulty is in the use of knowledge. A comprehensive theory does not provide either sufficient information or information structured in such a way that it can be used as the basis for practice. Additional information must be used; this is usually evident in case studies in which the interventions draw on information that is not included in the comprehensive theory.

Professions with a multiple-theories format do not have the same difficulties. What is at question for these professions is the definition of "theory." Not only do they not define theory as this text has, they usually do not define it at all. They see theory as a conceptual system that consists of information that can be directly applied to and/or includes information about application. In contrast, theory, as defined in Chapter 1 (page 7), is "an abstract description of a circumscribed set of physical phenomena that delineates the characteristics of the phenomena and their relationship to each other." These are not the same thing. Theory, in the context of a multiple-theories format, needs to be defined in such a way that it is evident how basic scientific inquiry is used to develop, refine, and test these conceptual systems.

One may be tempted to propose that some professions with a multiple-theories format, particularly those that have *theories-with-application*, seem to be moving towards a neopositivistic orientation. Perhaps it is only a matter of semantics that theories-with-application seem so similar to the "sets of guidelines for practice" of the neopositivistic orientation. However, equating them would not be a wise proposal because the difference between the two orientations is quite deep. It goes to the core of basic epistemological questions, to the nature of knowledge used in the professions, and to how that knowledge is developed, refined, and assessed.

Finally, the major disadvantage of the disciplinal orientation is that it does not draw upon the rich theoretical information contained within the bodies of knowledge of the various scientific disciplines. Similar to the traditional epistemological orientation, the disciplinal orientation is also in many ways without the cognitive capital of science (Merton, 1982).

The Neopositivistic Orientation

Positivism is a philosophical orientation that takes the position that knowledge derived from basic scientific inquiry can and should be used for the advancement of human ends. Positivists place basic science in an exalted position, seeing it as holding the solution to a majority of human problems. For the most part, positivism came to an abrupt end on August 6, 1945, when the atomic bomb was dropped on Hiroshima. It was replaced by neopositivism, a more tempered point of view. Neopositivism takes the position that knowledge derived from basic scientific inquiry is important and should be used in assisting humankind (Wulff, et al., 1986). However, such knowledge will not necessarily lead to the resolution of all problems, and limits should be put on its use. Ethical considerations in the use of scientific knowledge are recognized as essential.

The term *neopositivism* was selected as the label for this epistemological orientation for two reasons. First, it embodies the idea of using theoretical information for practical ends. Second, it implies recognition of the limits of theoretical information as the basis for practice. Practice is more than the application of theoretical information. It is a human endeavor, and there is art in practice.

The neopositivistic orientation is discussed only briefly here, drawing upon the work of Beckstrand, 1986; Collins and Fielder, 1986; Hardy, 1973; Mosey, 1981, 1986; Newman, 1986; and Schein, 1972. A more lengthy and detailed description is provided in the next section of the text. As its organization of knowledge is one of the key characteristics of this orientation, it is presented first.

Organization

In the neopositivistic orientation, the knowledge of a profession is considered to be on three levels:

I. *A Fundamental Body of Knowledge*—Viewed as basic to all of practice, it is made up of five categories of information:

A. Philosophical assumptions—the beliefs a profession holds about the nature of the individual, environment, and goals of the profession.

B. Ethical code—standards and principles of human conduct that serve as a guide for determining what is moral behavior in professional activities.

C. Theoretical foundation—theories and empirical data selected from appropriate disciplines that serve as the scientific base for practice.

D. Domain of concern—areas of human experience in which members of the profession have expertise and offer assistance to others.

E. Legitimate tools—those activities, instruments, modalities, methods, and processes in which members of a profession have expertise, and that they use as the media for assisting clients.

II. *An Applied Body of Knowledge*—Knowledge that is compatible with a profession's fundamental body of knowledge and serves as the basis for day-to-day practice, including:

A. Sets of guidelines for practice—internally consistent information extrapolated from theories or empirical data that provides direction for identifying and resolving those clinical problems that are within a profession's domain of concern.

B. Screening tools—procedures used for preliminary assessment.

III. *Practice*—Information basic to skilled and ethical use of a profession's applied body of knowledge for the purpose of collaborative problem identification and resolution with a client, including:

A. Aspects and sequence of practice.

B. Use of an applied body of knowledge.

C. Clinical reasoning and decision making.

D. The art of practice.

Applied Scientific Inquiry in the Health Professions

In a neopositivistic orientation, each profession's fundamental body of knowledge is made up of the five categories of knowledge outlined above, but the information included in each category varies from profession to profession.

Origin   Like the disciplinal orientation, the neopositivistic epistemological orientation has its origin in the dawning awareness that use of basic scientific knowledge will ultimately lead to more effective practice. Rational empiricism is also accepted as fundamental to scientific inquiry. Differences between the orientations are related to (a) beliefs held regarding the use of theoretical knowledge and (b) the source and organization of that knowledge.

In the neopositivistic orientation, theoretical knowledge is viewed as not directly applicable to practice. Moreover, theoretical knowledge is seen as generated by, and selected from, appropriate disciplines. There is no attempt to organize theoretical knowledge into a comprehensive theory; it remains unsystematized within the "theoretical foundation" category of the fundamental body of knowledge.

The source of a profession's fundamental body of knowledge, at least in the beginning, is the unstated traditions of the profession. What appears to happen over time is a sorting out, and articulation of, the content of the five categories. Philosophical assumptions, aspects of the domain of concern, and legitimate tools, for example, are separated from each other and clearly stated. This is a lengthy process and not without controversy. What were vague, tacit understandings may look quite different when clearly articulated and written down.

The theoretical foundation of a profession's fundamental body of knowledge may be the last to be clearly stated. It begins with identifying theoretical information that appears to be basic to practice. The content of the theoretical foundation becomes more specific and refined as the profession clarifies just exactly what theories and empirical data it uses in its sets of guidelines for practice.

The source of a profession's applied body of knowledge typically comes through examination of its collection of particular solutions for the theoretical support behind them. When support is found, and the particular solution is thought to be at least somewhat effective, it is reformulated into a set of guidelines for practice and subjected to formal assessment. In this process, many particular solutions are left behind because they are either ineffective or are replaced by sets of guidelines for practice. While some particular solutions may remain for a time as part of the profession's applied body of knowledge, most are replaced by sets of guidelines for practice. Dentistry is an example of a profession that has moved from particular solutions to sets of guidelines for practice. When dentistry had a traditional epistemological orientation, the particular solution for a serious toothache was to pull the tooth. Now dentistry has sets of guidelines for practice that help to identify possible causes and treatments for toothache. Pulling teeth has become the treatment of last resort. Like the articulation of a fundamental body of knowledge, developing an applied body of knowledge is a lengthy and controversial process.

Nature   The content of the fundamental body of knowledge of a given profession is unique in its totality, rather than in any one of its parts. For example, human anatomy is included in the theoretical foundation of many health professions, and edema is in the domain of concern of nursing, physical therapy, and occupational therapy. Although professions share aspects of their fundamental body of knowledge with other professions, taken in its totality each profession's fundamental body of knowledge is unique.

A neopositivistic orientation is pluralistic—the belief there is more than one basic principle, that everything cannot be reduced to a single principle (Wulff, Pedersen, & Rosenberg, 1986). Therefore, there are no dominant concepts or postulates. The five categories of a fundamental body of knowledge are considered to be of equal importance to the profession and to practice. One category does not govern another. Because their relationship is interdependent and dynamic, change in the content of one category often leads to change in other categories.

In the neopositivistic orientation, each profession has an applied body of knowledge made up primarily of sets of guidelines for practice. For each profession, the sets of guidelines differ in structure as well as content, according to need. For example, the sets of guidelines for practice of medicine, "diagnostic categories," are structured around signs and symptoms, pathology, etiology, prevention, treatment/management, course, and sequelae. In contrast, the sets of guidelines for practice of occupational therapy, "frames of reference," are structured around theoretical base, function/dysfunction continua, behaviors and physical signs indicative of function and dysfunction, and postulates regarding change.

The applied body of knowledge of each profession is unique, but occasionally sets of guidelines for practice may be shared. An example is the set of guidelines developed by Rood (1954) that is used by both physical and occupational therapists. Sets of guidelines for practice for different professions may look rather similar at first glance because they are founded on the same theoretical information—biomechanics or a particular learning theory, for example. A more detailed examination usually reveals their differences.

A word of caution: Sets of guidelines for practice are not theories. They are derived from theoretical information, but are very different than theories. They are sets of guidelines for practice and remain sets of guidelines for practice. They are not an entity that somehow becomes a theory. Nor does a theory ever become a set of guidelines for practice.

Ideology   In a neopositivistic orientation, ideology is contained within the category of *philosophical assumptions*. A profession's code of ethics should also be thought of as part of its ideology. Because ideology is separate from other components in this orientation, it can be studied both in its own right and in its relationship to the other categories of the fundamental body of knowledge, to the applied body of knowledge, to practice, and to society. Study involves use of the various methods of philosophical inquiry.

Form of Inquiry   The primary form of scientific inquiry in a neopositivistic orientation is applied. Sets of guidelines for practice are developed and refined, and their adequacy is assessed through applied Type I and Type II inquiry.

Use   The organization of knowledge described above is in part also a description of how knowledge is used in the neopositivistic orientation. The third level, practice, involves skilled and ethical use of the applied body of knowledge. Sets of guidelines for practice are chosen to assist in problem identification and problem resolution with a particular client. Judith Larsen (1981) refers to this as "instrumental utilization" in that the sets of guidelines and ultimately the theoretical information from which they are derived are evident, can be cited, and are able to be documented. This aspect of the neopositivistic orientation is discussed in more detail in Chapter 5. However, it should be noted at this point that "problem resolution" does not necessarily imply "solution." Rather, it refers to assisting a client to deal with a problem in a manner that is seen as beneficial by the client.

Comments

There are three major advantages to the neopositivistic orientation. First, it is quite specific about the relationship between theory and practice. The organization of knowledge into three levels defines the link between theoretical knowledge, application of theoretical knowledge, and daily work with clients. Second, it provides specific information about assessment and intervention relative to the various elements of a profession's domain of concern. Third, it makes use of the methods and research designs of science to (a) transform theoretical knowledge into information that can be used to resolve practical problems and (b) assess the adequacy of problem resolution.

However, the neopositivistic orientation has disadvantages that fall loosely into three categories: (a) tendency toward its inappropriate use and abuse, (b) reaction against its use, and (c) inherent problems.

Tendency Toward Inappropriate Use and Abuse

Argyris and Schon are two of the major critics of the neopositivistic orientation, focusing primarily on its inappropriate use and abuse (Argyris & Schon, 1974; Schon, 1983). Their first concern is the complacency of practitioners that is fostered by this orientation. In their opinion, sets of guidelines for practice are used out of habit or to maintain a profession's unquestioned world view or ideology. Sets of guidelines are not evaluated for effectiveness formally or informally. Neopositivism does not promote reflection on practice or the situation of practice. Complacency also leads to the use of sets of guidelines that are based on obsolete theoretical information. Once a set of guidelines for practice is formulated, the profession gives little attention to research findings related to the theoretical information fundamental to that set of guidelines. Complacency creates a false sense of security for the profession.

Second, Argyris and Schon are concerned about the relationship among sets of guidelines for practice, actual practice, and theoretical information. They feel practitioners frequently say they are using a given set of guidelines for practice when in actuality they are not. Practitioners may be using a different set of guidelines—for instance, claiming to use a neurologically based set of guidelines that is actually based on biomechanical principles—or they may be using no guidelines at all. Further, Argyris and Schon argue, many sets of guidelines are so poorly or incompletely stated that it is difficult to determine what, if any, theoretical information was used in their formulation.

Finally, Argyris and Schon are concerned about limitations in the way neopositivistic practitioners perceive their clients because they believe that the neopositivistic orientation defines problems and solutions outside of the context of the individual. If the problem of the client is inadequately or incorrectly defined, the solution is irrelevant. The situation may not be what it seems, and many important variables may be ignored. In the search for a rigorously stated set of guidelines, relevancy to practice is lost.

The criticism of Argyris and Schon regarding the neopositivistic orientation should be noted with care because what they say is quite true when this orientation is not used with understanding.

Reaction Against Use

Reaction against use of a neopositivistic orientation seems to be on two levels. One is philosophical, related to the issue of what science-based professions are, or should be (Beckstrand, 1986; Christiansen, 1990; Dickoff & James, 1968; Fitzpatrick & Whall, 1983; Fleming et al., 1987; Kielhofner, 1983). Some individuals, both within and outside of professions, believe that professions must become more like scientific disciplines to remain viable. They say attention should be focused on the development of theoretical knowledge unique to the profession. Only theoretical information developed by the profession should be considered legitimate as the basis for practice. Their objection to the neopositivistic orientation is that theoretical information selected from a variety of disciplines serves as the foundation for practice, and that is not good. While the reasoning behind this position is often not clearly stated, the implication seems to be that a profession without a self-developed theoretical body of knowledge is a technical, rather than science-based, occupation. Most, but not all, of the individuals taking the above position are most comfortable with the disciplinal orientation.

The other reaction against the use of the neopositivistic orientation focuses more on the level of practice. Some practitioners, particularly those whose professional education was not in this orientation, are uncomfortable using sets of guidelines for practice. They tend to find them restrictive, preferring a more intuitive approach. In working with clients who have multiple problems, they have difficulty with the idea that various sets of guidelines are used simultaneously or sequentially. Although these problems can be overcome through study and practice under adequate supervision, their concerns are still quite real.

Inherent Problems   There are some inherent problems in the neopositivistic orientation. One, identified by Schein (1972), is the conflict between the convergence of theoretical information and the divergence of practice. In categorizing phenomena and developing concepts, common elements are identified, while idiosyncratic characteristics or those considered irrelevant are ignored. Theoretical information, which is made up of concepts, accentuates similarities, causing the phenomena to converge. For example, in first studying human anatomy one learns about the parts of the body, where they are located, and so forth. One learns about the typical body, but the multiple differences between individual bodies are given little attention. Practice, on the other hand, highlights divergence. Each person is different in many ways, as is the situation of each person. Although the convergence/divergence issue is not resolved in the neopositivistic orientation, an attempt is made to deal with it through the flexibility inherent in sets of guidelines for practice that provide direction for problem identification and resolution, rather than rigid rules. Within limits, sets of guidelines for practice can be altered to meet the individual needs of clients.

Lack of adequate basic scientific knowledge is another problem in the neopositivistic orientation. There is so much that is unknown. At times adequate sets of guidelines for practice cannot be developed because of insufficient theoretical information. Practitioners sometimes work in the dark, feeling their way, using practical inquiry, hoping for the intuitive leap that will shed light. Practice at times is not supported by theoretical information. However, one of the hallmarks of the neopositivistic orientation is a cognizance of the lack of theoretical support and of the need to work continually with appropriate disciplines in the search for theoretical knowledge.

The third problem in the neopositivistic orientation is the use of applied scientific inquiry, both in developing sets of guidelines for practice and in assessing their adequacy. As mentioned in Chapter 1, our understanding of how practical knowledge is extrapolated from theoretical information is primitive at best. Our understanding of applied Type I inquiry is almost pre-Bacon—that is, comparable to the age before the dawn of modern basic science. This problem does not negate the usefulness of a neopositivistic orientation, but it may impede the development of sets of guidelines for practice.

On the other hand, there is some understanding of applied Type II inquiry concerned with assessment of the adequacy of sets of guidelines for practice. With that understanding, however, is an awareness of how difficult it is to evaluate effectiveness and efficiency of sets of guidelines for practice. Individual differences are legion and many variables cannot be controlled. Gaining the cooperation of a sufficient number of participants is also difficult. Cost in time and money hardly needs to be mentioned. Moreover, evaluative findings can usually only be stated in terms of probability (Wulff, Pedersen, & Rosenberg, 1986)—that is, we can only say that use of a particular set of guidelines for practice is likely to be effective X percent of the time. There is no way of determining whether the use of a given set of guidelines will be effective in assisting a particular individual.

Difficulties with assessing adequacy relative to intervention or treatment is a problem in all of the epistemological orientations described in this chapter.

The Phenomenological Orientation

Phenomenology, a school of philosophy, considers phenomena as the only objects of knowledge or as the only form of reality (Greene, 1973; Phillips, 1987; Singleton, et al., 1988; Wulff, Pedersen, & Rosenberg, 1986). Phenomena are observable entities—persons, nonhuman things, and events. Phenomenologists believe that phenomena should be studied as individual entities in and of themselves, in their entirety, but not as part of a collectivity. The development of general principles or theories, therefore, is not considered the proper goal of scientific inquiry. A person, for example, can only be understood in terms of his or her *particular* anatomy, physiology, attitudes, feelings, values, motives, and past and current life situation.

Understanding—or subjective knowledge—is the cornerstone of phenomenalism, as opposed to objective knowledge, which describes, explains, and makes predictions about phenomena. Understanding is gained through reflection—casting back, pondering, carefully considering, deliberating (Flexner & Hauck, 1987). Reflection may take place in the immediacy of interaction with phenomena, after interaction, or both (Schon, 1983). When individuals are part of the phenomena, their perceptions, beliefs and assigned meanings constitute the essence of the situation. The "observer" or outsider who wishes to understand must suspend his or her ways of perceiving in order to comprehend the situation. However, one cannot truly be an outside observer; being part of the situation changes the self and the situation. Thus, one must not only reflect on the situation of others, but also be self-reflective. Reflection is a continuous process because no situation is ever static.

Phenomenalism is often compared and contrasted with rational empiricism, as was done to some extent in the above paragraphs. Indeed, phenomenalism developed in part as a reaction to rational empiricism. The reductionistic and mechanistic aspects of rational empiricism were considered impediments to gaining "true" knowledge, particularly knowledge of the individual. However, phenomenalism should not be seen only as a response to rational empiricism because it is an important philosophical school of thought in its own right.

Phenomenologists take various positions regarding rational empiricism, from viewing it as an unacceptable or irrelevant means of gaining knowledge to considering it as one among several ways of gaining knowledge. The latter group considers biological, psychological, and sociological theories as legitimate knowledge that serves to describe the objective situation of the individual. But such knowledge is considered to be inadequate because it is only partial. Phenomenologists use theoretical knowledge as a backdrop for understanding—a backdrop, however, that can be easily ignored.

Argyris and Schon have described an epistemological orientation to practice that they refer to as "reflection-in-action" but have not identified it as being part of any broader epistemological category (Argyris & Schon, 1974; Schon, 1983). Because this idea seems so firmly grounded in phenomenalism, it, as well as the work of Foss and Rothenberg (1987), will be used as the basis for discussion of the phenomenological orientation.

Origin   Like phenomenalism in general, the origin of the phenomenological orientation to practice seems to be a reaction to a previously dominant school of thought—in this case, to the neopositivistic orientation. Many of the factors leading to that reaction were described earlier as disadvantages of the neopositivistic orientation, particularly those listed under "tendency toward inappropriate use and abuse" (see page 34).

Proponents of the phenomenological orientation view the circumstances of practice as uncertain, unstable, unique to the individual or situation, and prone to value conflicts. Much of practice involves dealing with problem situations for which there are no sets of guidelines for practice and no theoretical knowledge. Thus, they believe that a new epistemology of practice is called for—one that addresses the fluid circumstances of practice.

Nature   In the phenomenological orientation, knowledge is considered to be primarily tacit and implicit rather than explicit. Knowledge is revealed *in* action as opposed to articulated *before* action. It is the "kind of knowing that does not stem from a prior intellectual operation" (Flexner & Hauck, 1987, p. 1002). To a great extent, it is intuitive—the immediate apprehension of an idea, fact, or truth, independent of any reasoning process.

Emphasis is placed on the *art of practice*. The term "art" means in this context "skill in conducting any human activity." Art is seen as essential in dealing with the uncertainty and uniqueness of individual situations that are found in practice. Practice is viewed as the setting for the doing of art—the atelier. Schon (1983) specifically equates the work of the practitioner with that of the artist.

Delineation of a client's problems and how they might be resolved is referred to as "theory." Although they have the same label, the theory of phenomenology and the theory of rational empiricism are not the same. For the phenomenologist, theory is a description of a unique case. It deals with a narrow range of particular and present phenomena and is not meant for generalization beyond that one case. In rational empiricism, theory is not particular to a single individual, situation, event, or thing. It is concerned with categories of phenomena and may be generalized to all specific phenomena contained within those categories. It is not time specific. (Rational empiricism will be discussed in more detail later.)

Basic ideas about the nature of theory, its structure, and purpose are very different for phenomenologists and rational empiricists. To minimize confusion, "unique-case theory" will be used in this book in relation to the phenomenological orientation, and "theory" will be used in relation to rational empiricism and, by extension, the disciplinal and neopositivistic orientations.

Ideology
The phenomenological orientation gives little attention to the goals and boundaries of a profession. These are considered givens, known to practitioners. Beliefs about the individual and the environment are described by practitioners, however. The individual and his or her environment are seen as unique. No two clients or client situations are the same. Such a view goes far beyond the simple recognition of individual differences and is essential to understanding the ideology of this epistemological orientation.

Form of Inquiry
In the phenomenological orientation, inquiry takes place in the immediacy of practice within the context of each case. "Immediacy" refers to the time one is with a client or thinking about clients. Inquiry and assisting a client are intimately connected; one cannot be easily separated from the other.

One comes to understand a client through observation and questioning. The practitioner attempts to remain naive, inhibiting personal biases, preconceived ideas, and categorization. One listens and experiences the data, making them a part of one's self. The immediate purpose is to make sense of the situation from the client's point of view; the ultimate purpose is to assist a client in identifying his or her problems and their resolution. Reflection is the primary method of inquiry, with intuition and problem solving also playing an important role.

What has just been described is the process of developing, refining, and testing a *unique-case theory*. A unique-case theory delineates the characteristics of the client, his or her current life situation, the client's problems, and what the practitioner and client did to resolve these problems. Thus, a unique-case theory is not "complete" until the end of intervention.

Organization   The phenomenological orientation to practice seems to have one level of knowledge—"unique-case theory." Yet the question remains as to what exactly is the body of knowledge in the phenomenological orientation. What constitutes a profession's body of knowledge? What are its constituent parts? These questions can be answered in four different ways:

Using a very narrow interpretation, the phenomenological orientation holds that there is no substantial body of knowledge. Knowledge is ephemeral, short-lived, and transitory. In the context of a unique-case theory, when intervention with a client is ended the knowledge dissipates. A unique-case theory is never applied again because it is specific to a client in a given situation. This would ensure that the practitioner would come to practice with the necessary degree of naivete. However, this interpretation is hardly ever contemplated by a profession because, if it were taken one step further, it would mean that anyone would be able to practice in any profession.

A second way of responding to these questions is to say that a profession's body of knowledge is conceptualized as discrete units of information in the form of case studies, examples, protocols, precedents, and the like. These units are not ordered in any discernable way. The body of knowledge acts as a pool out of which each unique-case theory is devel-

Figure 2. A summary of four epistemological orientations to practice: traditional, disciplinal, neopositivistic, and phenomenological.

	Traditional	Disciplinal	Neopositivistic	Phenomenological
Origin of Knowledge	From what was done in the past	Rational empiricism; Philosophy of basic scientific inquiry	Rational empiricism; Neopositivism; Philosophy of applied scientific inquiry	Reaction to neopositivism; Phenomenological school of philosophy
Nature of Knowledge	Particular solution for each problem	Comprehensive theory or multiple theories	Theoretically-based sets of guidelines for practice	"Unique-case theory"
Ideology of Profession	Not consciously considered	Intertwined with comprehensive theory; Unclear relative to multiple theories	Treated as separate from scientific knowledge	Relative to individual/environment, rather than goals of profession; No relationship to scientific information as such; not considered important
Form of Inquiry	Generally not encouraged; Practical inquiry	Basic scientific inquiry	Applied scientific inquiry	Reflection
Organization of Knowledge	One level: practice	One level: fundamental body of knowledge	Three levels: fundamental body of knowledge, applied body of knowledge, practice	One level: practice
Use of Knowledge	Use accepted means of solving a problem	Comprehensive theory/multiple theories serve as a way of thinking about practice, a context for action	Selected sets of guidelines for practice used alone, in combination, or sequentially	Knowledge is not "used" but rather created anew in the process of assisting each client

oped. However, this way of viewing knowledge would interfere with the desired practitioner naivete, causing a conflict between knowing the body of knowledge yet not bringing preconceived ideas to practice.

The third possible type of organization is that which was found in the disciplinal orientation. The knowledge of the profession is organized within the structure of a comprehensive theory. This theory serves as the backdrop for the development of unique-case theories, but it also creates the same naivete/knowledge conflict. Moreover, a disciplinal orientation is based primarily on rational empiricism. Since phenomenalism and rational empiricism are not really compatible with each other, ignoring this conflict is likely to lead to a split between the comprehensive theory and unique-case theories.

The fourth possible type of organization is a combination of the second and third, resulting in a three-tier organizational structure: a comprehensive theory, discrete units of descriptive information, and unique-case theories. While this does seem to be a possibility, from an epistemological perspective it is a bit of a mess.

Use

The idea of "use of knowledge" is not well-suited to discussion of the phenomenological orientation. Phenomenologists do not think in terms of using knowledge because of the intermingling of knowing and doing—of inquiry and practice. A unique-case theory is developed in the process of interacting with a client in the context of the client's situation. Knowledge is not completely developed until the end of the practitioner-client interaction. Then, being ephemeral, it is quickly gone. Phenomenalists do not *use* knowledge; instead, knowledge is created in action and, in a sense, *is* the action.

Comments

There are three advantages to a phenomenological orientation to practice. First, it is client- and client/situation-centered. The focus is on gaining an understanding from the perspective of the client. It emphasizes the specialness of the individual and the vast variety of individual and situational differences. Second, the phenomenological orientation highlights the dangers of bringing preconceived ideas, set categories, and personal and professional biases to practice. Such intellectual baggage may lead to inattention to clients' needs, misperception of clients' problems, and the improper imposition of one's own values on clients. The third advantage of the phenomenological orientation is its focus on the importance of reflection—thinking about what one is doing and what happens in the client-practitioner interaction. Attention to the process of reflection—making reflection a conscious part of daily practice—minimizes any tendencies toward the mechanization of practice. Reflection is one of the cornerstones of good practice, regardless of epistemological orientation.

The major disadvantage of the phenomenological orientation is its lack of a defined body of knowledge. While it is well and good to be attentive to the client, to understand how the client perceives the problem at hand, and to have common agreement between client and practitioner regarding goals, what then does one do? If the practitioner has no more knowledge than the client, why has the client sought help from the practitioner? The practitioner's ability to engage in reflective thinking, to observe, question, and problem solve would seem to be for nought without some body of knowledge to draw from. It would be like asking someone who has absolutely no idea how bread looks, tastes, or is made to make a loaf.

The various kinds of bodies of knowledge that are sometimes included in a phenomenological orientation are just that—*sometimes* included. They are not central to the orientation and often are not even mentioned. Some of the questions basic to the epistemology of practice do not seem to be satisfactorily addressed in the phenomenological orientation. The problem with making this statement is the lack of consensus regarding what questions should be addressed in an epistemology of practice. The author's bias towards the neopositivistic orientation has influenced what questions are selected, how they are stated, and what the criteria are for a reasonable answer. The problems identified in the phenomenological orientation, as well as the disciplinal orientation, may well be the result of the wrong questions being asked.

As an observer of practice, it seems to me that phenomenalism has had the greater influence on the health professions as a philosophical school of thought, as opposed to an epistemological orientation to practice. The advantages of this orientation—client-centered practice, for instance—have become part of the ideology of many professions that do not in any way subscribe to a phenomenological epistemology of practice.

In conclusion, four epistemological orientations to practice have been identified. Although each has been described as distinct, many professions combine two or more epistemological orientations. However, there are problems in doing so because the four epistemological orientations are not compatible with each other in many ways. Each says something quite different about knowledge fundamental to practice and, by extension, about science-based professions in general. When a profession uses more than one epistemological orientation, it tends to have difficulty identifying, developing, and describing its own body of knowledge and stating how that body of knowledge is used in practice. To an outsider, such professions seem to be unfocused and inarticulate, especially relating to the area of scientific inquiry. A single, specifically stated epistemological orientation to practice is very useful to a profession and is likely to facilitate its continued growth and effectiveness.

Section II:
Neopositivistic Orientation in More Detail

This section provides a description of the neopositivistic orientation to practice in greater depth and detail. Structurally, it follows the organization of knowledge of this orientation: fundamental body of knowledge, applied body of knowledge, and practice.

3. *Fundamental Body of Knowledge*

A profession's fundamental body of knowledge is a compilation all of the information a profession recognizes as basic to, and supportive of, its applied body of knowledge and practice. The information is typically a combination of philosophical and scientific knowledge drawn from a variety of sources. It may also include some practical knowledge.

The content of a profession's fundamental body of knowledge consists of five categories of information: philosophical assumptions, ethical code, theoretical foundation, domain of concern, and legitimate tools. The categories form a simple taxonomy developed to organize the considerable and diverse knowledge base of professions. They were formed by the author after surveying health profession literature to identify types of knowledge shared by the majority of professions (Mosey, 1981; 1986). The categories seemed to account for most types of information with little loss of knowledge or overlap between categories. Because of this good fit, and with full recognition of the limitations of any taxonomy, this system will be used to describe the fundamental body of knowledge of professions.

While the specific knowledge contained within each category differs to a great extent for each profession, there is some shared knowledge, which is to be expected in a group of professions concerned with a common area such as health. The overlap of knowledge is also very useful because it facilitates understanding and communication that, in turn, tends to enhance our ability to assist clients.

Introduction

The origins of most professions are not really known. What seems to happen is that a process begins in which society identifies an unfulfilled need, and people who believe they can satisfy that need come together to assist society in that area. Eventually these people move from being an occupational group to a profession when a fundamental body of knowledge evolves and becomes increasingly larger, more refined, and of greater complexity.[1]

Over a period of time, a profession's fundamental body of knowledge comes to be codified in some way. The first textbooks are written, and the profession begins to describe itself in more detail to the wider community. Four factors seem to influence this process. The first is movement of education for the profession from primarily on-site apprenticeships to academic settings. Academic education demands a fairly well-articulated fundamental body of knowledge. A second factor is society's need to know what is fundamental to a profession's expertise. Professions cannot exist without the support of society. To gain such support a profession must be able to articulate its rationale, goals, and means in a manner understandable to members of society. The third factor is when a profession asks itself: "What is our knowledge base?" It is the attempt to answer this question that, in part, motivates a profession to study and codify its fundamental body of knowledge. The fourth factor, closely related to the third, is a profession's need for a collective identity—an identity that differentiates it from all other professions. Although a profession establishes its identity through a variety of means, one method is by articulating a fundamental body of knowledge.

At some point in the evolution of a profession, the profession and its fundamental body of knowledge are joined. The profession comes to define itself by its fundamental body of knowledge. This is particularly evident relative to a profession's domain of concern. For example, the physical therapist is called for gait training, a dentist for a toothache, a social worker for assistance with a nursing home placement. The pro-

---

[1] Many of the ideas in this section are drawn from the work of Dingwall (1982), Etzioni (1969), Goodlad (1984), Hughes (1973), M. S. Larsen (1977), McGlothlin (1964), Moore (1970), J. C. Rogers (1983), Schein (1972), and Wollmer and Mills (1966).

fession has a sense of knowing what it is about. This is not to say that what a profession believes and does are always congruent with the perceptions of those outside of the profession.

The fundamental body of knowledge of a profession is never static; it is dynamic and continually changing. This characteristic maintains the viability of a profession over time. Change may be quite slow and barely noticeable or very rapid and almost revolutionary. The latter is illustrated by the changes in psychiatry following the introduction of psychotropic drugs. There are many factors that lead to change in a profession's fundamental body of knowledge, including:

The creation of new or refined theoretical knowledge.

Professions have the responsibility of monitoring the development of theoretical knowledge that is potentially relevant to their domain of concern, selecting what is appropriated, and incorporating that information into their theoretical foundation. An example of this is the inclusion of various learning theories into the theoretical foundation of many of the health professions. However, there is often a lag between the creation of knowledge and the recognition of its importance to a profession. A classic example is the delay between Flemings's identification of the interaction between some types of bacteria and a substance produced by a particular mold—which he named penicillin—in 1928 and the incorporation of this knowledge into medicine's theoretical foundation in the early 1940s (Perutz, 1989).

In addition, professions request development of theoretical knowledge from appropriate disciplines, especially when available information is not adequate for resolving a particular problem. The knowledge requested about and developed with regard to the immune system that was subsequently used to enhance recipient acceptance of organ transplants is an example.

The needs of society.

Society may identify a new need or may demand assistance with a need heretofore given little attention. The former is exemplified by the acquired immune deficiency syndrome (AIDS), the latter by rehabilitation of individuals with traumatic brain injury (TBI).

When a need is identified, society seeks assistance from various professions. Additional information must often be added to the fundamental body of knowledge of the responding professions in order for their assistance to be effective.

A shift in the values, beliefs, and priorities of society.

Such a shift can take many forms, such as the demand for more openness on the part of practitioners, the concern about equitable allocation of money for health care, and the ethical issues surrounding dying and death. Such shifts often lead to changes in the philosophical assumptions and the codes of ethics of professions.

Since the five categories that constitute a fundamental body of knowledge are interrelated, change in the content of one category frequently leads to change in the content of other categories. For example, when a new area of human experience is added to a profession's domain of concern, there are, almost by necessity, additions to the profession's theoretical foundation. Continuous alteration in content requires professions to attend to the synchrony of content between categories, making adjustments where needed. For instance, when a new moral principle (see page 60) is added to a profession's code of ethics, the profession examines its philosophical assumptions to determine whether they are congruent with the new principle and then makes changes in one or more of the assumptions, if necessary.

As professions add new content to their fundamental bodies of knowledge, so must they delete outdated content. Many professions have trouble deleting content due either to some need to hold on to tradition, or simply to inattention to the process of deletion. In fact, one of the major criticisms of professions by disciplines is that a significant part of the information included in the theoretical foundation of many professions—that which appears in curricula and textbooks—was demonstrated to be invalid some time ago or has been replaced by more refined and valid information (Glazer, 1980; Lieb, 1986).

Evolution of a profession's fundamental body of knowledge is not unbounded. Even when change is rapid and considerable, there are a variety of con-

Applied Scientific Inquiry in the Health Professions

straints that temper the degree and kind of change. The professions themselves tend to be conservative, tradition bound, and leery of new ideas. Any major change may be suspect and requires lengthy discussion in a struggle between the old guard and young Turks. However, such conflict may be very useful in invigorating a profession.

A profession's fundamental body of knowledge serves as a more specific constraint to change. Acting as a filter, it is instrumental in the selection and rejection of knowledge for inclusion. Questions—such as: Does this knowledge fit? Is it compatible with the philosophy of the profession? Is it congruent with the profession's domain of concern?— are addressed by comparing the new knowledge with the existing fundamental body of knowledge. Information considered far outside of the sphere of a profession's fundamental body of knowledge is usually not accepted for inclusion. The screening function of a fundamental body of knowledge and that of the comprehensive theory of the disciplinal orientation are different in degree rather than kind. The filter has much larger openings—allowing more new information in—in the neopositivistic orientation than in the disciplinal orientation.

The third constraint to change is a profession's hesitancy to engage in problem identification and resolution in areas of human experience in which it does not have sufficient knowledge and skill. A responsible profession does not attempt to enter a new area without first determining that a sufficient portion of its members have developed the appropriate expertise and understanding, because such a movement could be harmful to clients. In addition, promising much more than can be delivered may ultimately be detrimental to the reputation of the profession. Movement into a new area may be instigated by a small cadre of a profession's members or may be encouraged by society in general; in either case, a wise profession moves with caution.

A fourth constraint on the evolution of professions is their tendency to be possessive of the content of their fundamental bodies of knowledge. This is reflected in state licensure laws that, at least in part, are designed to protect a profession's "territory" from other professions. The most jealously guarded areas seem to be the domain of concern and legitimate tools. On the positive side, territorial conflicts help the professions to refine and clarify their fundamental bodies of knowledge.

The final constraint on change is the society to which the profession is responsible. To a great extent, society negotiates the differing responsibilities of each profession through a continuing dialogue. Accountability is a key factor in this dialogue. Society asks for assistance in various areas and ultimately demands evidence of successful rendering of services. A profession, in turn, defines its area of expertise and attempts to demonstrate a high degree of successful problem resolution. It is around these issues that negotiations occur. Society usually only supports a profession in those areas in which it believes the profession is effective.

Having outlined some of the general characteristics of a fundamental body of knowledge, specific attention is turned to the five categories of knowledge contained therein.

Philosophical Assumptions

A profession's philosophical assumptions are the basic beliefs it holds about the nature of the individual, the environment, the relationship between the individual and the environment, and the purpose and goals of the profession relative to meeting the needs of society. Philosophical assumptions are beliefs held to be "true," self-evident, and fundamental. In a metaphysical system, philosophical assumptions are the first premises of the system, serving as a foundation for development of the system. As givens in the logical process, what follows in the reasoning process only makes sense, if one accepts the first premises.

An example of a philosophical assumption is found in the United States' Declaration of Independence: "We hold these Truths to be self-evident, that all Men are created equal, that they are endowed by their Creator with certain inalienable Rights." These beliefs served as the basis for what follows in the document, a reasoned argument for self-government.

The philosophical assumptions of a profession are often used as the point of departure for reasoning as well as action. For example, a philosophical assumption from occupational therapy is: "Each individual has the right to seek his or her potential through personal choice within the context of some social constraints" (Mosey, 1986, p. 6).

Once an assumption is accepted by a profession, it is held with a fairly high degree of conviction and certainty and tends to be taken for granted. An assumption is only questioned when the profession is faced with extraordinary external events or when someone in the profession expresses strong doubts about one or several assumptions of the profession and has the ability to direct the profession's attention to examine and alter its assumptions.

The nature of the phenomena addressed by philosophical assumptions and scientific statements is different. Philosophical assumptions are concerned with abstract phenomena, scientific statements with physical phenomena. Their modes of inquiry are also different. For example, "all Men are created equal" is a philosophical statement referring to the belief that no person is preordained to govern by virtue of supernatural authority, economic advantage, skin color, or country of origin. While many would accept this as a philosophical assumption, few would accept it as a scientific statement. Both cursory observation and scientific data demonstrate that all people are not created equal in any number of ways—for instance, in terms of intelligence, longevity, emotional stability, and so forth. Confusion between philosophical assumptions and scientific statements sometimes leads to problems for a profession. A profession, for example, may attempt to deal with a philosophical issue or statement as if it could be subjected to scientific inquiry. Adequate investigation and sound decision making are unlikely to follow.

The philosophical assumptions of a profession may address many issues, but, in one way or another, most deal with the areas—the individual, the environment, and the goals of the profession—outlined in the definition. In regard to the individual, professions have many different perspectives and hold a number of different beliefs. Varying positions may be taken; the individual may be seen as self-determining, capable of making sound judgments, a free agent, rational, responsible, a partner. On the other hand, the individual may be viewed as in need of care and guidance and as being without the capacity to make any serious decisions regarding intervention.

Orientation to the practice environment also differs among professions. The environment may be narrowly defined as family or, more broadly, as extending to friends, community, and society as a whole. The components of the environment may be primarily people, or may also include (a) cultural beliefs, values and expectations and/or (b) the nonhuman, physical environment.

Positions differ regarding the degree to which the environment shapes the individual versus the degree to which the individual shapes the environment. Problems may be viewed as being primarily within the individual or as located mostly in the environment. For example, one might view homeless people as lacking the ability to find and hold jobs. Conversely, one may identify the economic situation as the primary cause of homelessness. Professions differ with regard to how they believe the environment can be used in problem resolution. On the other hand, the individual and the environment may be seen as so joined and interactive that no meaningful distinction can be made.

Lastly, philosophical assumptions are concerned with the purpose and goals of a profession. The purpose and goals may be seen as singular or multiple. Professions state their purposes and goals in a variety of ways; they may be quite general or very specific. They may focus on dysfunction/illness resolution or promotion of function/health. Some statements of purpose and goals include an overview of the profession's domain of concern, the population served, and a list of legitimate tools. The purpose and goals of a profession most clearly differentiate it from others.

While health professions would be expected to have differences in their philosophical assumptions, particularly in relation to purpose and goals, they tend to have some in common with regard to individuals and their environments. The philosophical assumption of occupational therapy, stated at the beginning of the section, is probably one of the assumptions of several other health professions. The commonality of assumptions across the professions would be expected because of the shared concern with health/illness/disability and our common evolution within Western society. Common assumptions promote mutual understanding and, thus, the likelihood of cooperative efforts.

Some philosophical assumptions may be the oldest part of a profession's fundamental body of knowledge. Many professions began with only a set of beliefs and some practical knowledge. These early statements about a profession's world view and reason for being are sometimes still evident in the profession's present-day assumptions. However, one may have to look closely to find them because the words used in stating an assumption often go through many changes.

The original assumptions of a profession tend to reflect one or more of the various schools of philosophy current at the time of the profession's origin. They also reflect the cultural belief of the society in which the profession was founded. This is exemplified by the influence of early 19th century humanitarianism on the philosophical assumptions of social work. As the profession evolves, additional philosophical assumptions are incorporated. Often these are the beliefs of various individuals seen as major contributors to the field. Rapid social change may lead a profession to review its philosophical assumptions and force it to add and delete assumptions to bring the profession more in line with a society's ideology. If the philosophical assumptions of a profession were incompatible with the beliefs of society, it is unlikely that society would seek assistance from the profession. Because the philosophical assumptions of a profession tend to contain beliefs and ideas from different times, schools of philosophy, and cultures, some assumptions may not be compatible with others. Professions tend be unaware of or ignore this dissonance. Rigorous philosophical inquiry regarding assumptions is usually not a high priority for a profession.

Philosophical assumptions are ideals. The degree of professional conformity to them is closely related to whether an assumption is (a) realistic and/or (b) truly generally accepted by members of the profession. Some assumptions may be neither. Thus, the assumptions actually operant in a profession may not be those that are stated. Instead, the profession primarily acts within a set of implicit assumptions. This lack of match between what a profession says it believes and what it does may be confusing to students, troubling to society, and may ultimately lead to cynicism in the profession.

Finally, some stated philosophical assumptions

may be more platitudes than real operating principles; they sound nice for public consumption but have no real meaning to the profession. For example, everyone in the health professions talks about such ideas as "quality of life" or "holistic," and they have quickly appeared in the philosophical assumptions of various professions. Faddish assumptions tend to disappear almost as rapidly as they appear.

Codes of Ethics   The ethical code of a profession is a statement of those standards and principles of conduct that serve as a guide for determining what is moral behavior in professional activities (Beauchamp & Childress,1983; Veatch, 1989).

On an abstract level, the study of ethics is a part of philosophy and theology. These disciplines are concerned with investigating and contemplating such matters as what is right and wrong, the meaning and nature of moral choices, and whether moral principles are discovered or are a human construct (Veatch, 1989; Wulff et al., 1986). Ultimately, philosophers and theologians concerned with ethics articulate moral principles—statements that may serve as a guide for determining what actions, or categories of actions, are morally required, prohibited, or permitted.

Consideration and use of ethical principles in decision making is usually only required when a contemplated act has moral significance (Childress, 1989; Hansen, 1989). Such an act is one in which an individual's actions will affect the rights of other individuals, the institutions of society, and/or the physical, mental, or moral development of the individual. Whether or not an act has moral significance depends upon the situation surrounding the act. For instance, in the ordinary course of events the decision to take a hot shower is not an act of moral significance, but it may become morally significant if there is a severe shortage of water or energy.

The need for ethical principles is most apparent when there is an "ethical dilemma"—that is, no obvious, agreed-upon, right course of action. In such a case, various options must be studied, and each option considered in the light of ethical principles (Brody, 1988).

The ethical codes of health professions and their

use in practice are often referred to as *applied ethics* (Veatch, 1989). They are not the abstract ethical principles of philosophers and theologians but, rather, are based on these principles. Moreover, they are considered to be applied because they are concerned with the knowledge, activities, and customs of a particular sphere of life—health, illness, disability, and death—in the health professions.

The codes of ethics of health professions are part of a broad category of applied ethics, most often referred to as "bioethics" (Veatch, 1989). Bioethics is the analysis of choices in issues related to (a) health care, (b) scientific inquiry that involves the use of human participants and animals, and (c) manipulation of genetic material. Bioethics is the concern of everyone.

The purpose or functions of a code of ethics are:

1. To articulate members' general position on broad moral issues related to the work of the profession.

2. To serve as a means of communicating what is commonly expected of members of the profession to peers, other professions, and consumers of its services.

3. To provide guidance in making ethical choices.

4. To express professionwide standards that are used as the basis for quality assurance and peer discipline within the profession.

5. To serves as a device to protect the profession against regulation by outside parties.

6. To give members a sense of common commitment in matters of principle that, in turn, contributes to the identity and integrity of the profession (Edwards & Graber, 1988).

The origin of the tradition of codes of ethics in the health profession is usually considered to be derived from the Hippocratic Oath (Veatch, 1989). This oath, describing the duties and obligations of physicians, comes out of an ancient school of medicine centered on the Greek Island of Cos in the 5th century BC. The acknowledged leader of this group was Hippocrates. The Hippocratic oath is now considered more a symbolic than a useful document for guiding ethical practice in medicine. However, three ethical principles still in common use are derived from this document: (a) to do no harm, (b) to act only within the limits of one's abilities, and (c) to protect the confidentiality of the client.

The codes of ethics of medicine and other health professions have evolved to meet the needs of the professions and the society that they serve. The more rapid changes in codes of ethics in the last 15 years or so are influenced by at least two major factors: (a) changes in society's values and norms regarding what is considered to be appropriate ethical behavior on the part of members of professions and (b) new knowledge and technological products which create previously unexamined ethical questions.

The moral positions of a profession are typically stated in a formal code of ethics that includes a preamble of some sort, a list of principles, and interpretive statements elaborating on each principle. The ethical thinking of a profession is also reflected in decisions made in disciplinary rulings, in official papers of the association representing the profession, and in essays written by members regarding various ethical questions (Hansen, 1988).

The content of codes of ethics has been categorized in a number of different ways. The two major categories used here are "moral principles" and "issues." Admittedly, there is some overlap between the two areas. The content described is an overview; one or more aspects may not be included in the code of ethics of a given profession. The enumeration is not meant to imply a ranking of value.

Moral Principles
(Childress, 1989)

1. Beneficence/Nonmaleficence—to confer benefit, not to do harm.

2. Utility—the net balance of an action is on the side of benefit over harm.

3. Respect for person—recognition of the autonomy of the individual; respect for the wishes of a competent person or his or her representative.

4. Truthfulness—honesty with a client or his or her representative, recognition of the right to informed consent, honesty in reporting status of clients and services rendered.

5. Fidelity—keeping promises and contracts.

6. Confidentiality—recognition of the right to privacy.

7. Justice—when choices need to be made, ben-

efits and harms are distributed fairly.

8. Universality—similar cases are treated in similar ways irrespective of an individual's race, creed, national origin, sex, age, religion, sexual orientation, handicap, social status, or financial situation.

Issues Addressed in Codes of Ethics (American Occupational Therapy Association, 1988; Capron, 1989; Hull, 1988)

1. Delivery of competent service by maintaining, accurately representing, and acting within one's area of expertise.

2. Compliance with federal and state laws and regulations.

3. Balancing the interests of individual clients and those of society.

4. Reporting incompetent, illegal, or unethical actions of others.

5. Accountability for one's judgments and actions.

6. Responsibility for the education of students.

7. Education of members of other professions and the public regarding the services of the profession.

8. Responsibility for improving the health care of the public.

9. Establishing, maintaining, and improving the standards of the profession.

10. Advancing the knowledge of the profession.

11. Adhering to standards regarding scientific inquiry involving human participants and animals.

12. Fair remuneration for services.

Although there are a number of difficulties with codes of ethics in the health professions, only a few will be touched on here (Edwards & Graber, 1988; Graber & Thomasma, 1989; Hull, 1988). First, there is the question of when, and to whom, do ethical codes apply. Since the codes are usually developed under the auspices of a national professional association, do they apply to individuals who do not elect to be members of the association? And, regardless of membership, what is the relationship between a profession's code of ethics and a member's personal code of ethics? Under what circumstances does one code have priority over the other? Many codes of ethics state that one must obey federal and state laws and regulations, yet acting outside the law is sometimes considered to be an acceptable way of challenging the law—as in the recent cases of physician-assisted death.

Second, many professions are not clear about which aspects of their code of ethics are to be treated as rules and which as guidelines. Rules spell out what conduct is considered acceptable, with the stricture that non-compliance or violation can lead to disciplinary procedures. Guidelines, on the other hand, are principles used to assist the practitioner in making moral choices; they are not binding.

Third, codes of ethics tend to lack internal consistencies, often putting one principle in conflict with another. Such a situation is exemplified in the tension between confidentiality and the need to give information to others in order to enhance the care of a client. Another potential conflict exists between the principle of universality and the lack of sufficient money to adequately treat all patients.

Fourth, in considering various ethical dilemmas, codes of ethics tend to be silent about which principles should be adapted, how they should be interpreted, which have priority, or how much weight should be accorded to what principles. What is often missing from codes of ethics and accompanying documents, if there are any, is information about how the code of ethics is used in practical situations. They say nothing about how to engage in the process of moral reasoning. In other words, codes rarely include information about ethical schools of thought or "theories" that can or should be used, alone or in combination, to consider moral questions (Childress, 1989). (This is the theoria of philosophy, not the theory of science.) There are many ethical theories, however; they are often categorized by the element of the dilemma that is considered most important in considering what action to take:

1. The motivation of the agent (virtue).
2. The act itself, or the means (deontological).
3. The immediate goal, or ends of the action (teleological).
4. The ultimate consequence, or effect of the action (consequentialist).

Applied Scientific Inquiry in the Health Professions

Finally, codes of ethics may identify issues or include statements that are not really related to what is considered to be a matter of ethical concern. Some codes of ethics do include precepts that seem more concerned with promoting or preserving the customs and or interests of the profession rather than the well-being of society (Hull, 1988). The prohibition against advertisement, once included in medicine's code of ethics, is a classic example.

Codes of ethics, like the other categories of knowledge included in a profession's fundamental body of knowledge, need to be reexamined regularly. More importantly, perhaps, members of professions need to become conversant in using their code of ethics in daily practice.

Theoretical Foundation

The theoretical foundation of a profession consists of selected theories and empirical data that serve as the scientific base for practice. Theoretical information is drawn from those disciplines that study phenomena of concern to the profession, typically the biological and social sciences.

The theoretical foundations of allied health professions usually also contain information from the applied body of knowledge of medicine. As the various health professions deal with problems related to illness, they need information contained within diagnostic categories. What information they need is dependent on the particular profession. For example, the information needed by nursing may be somewhat different than the information needed by rehabilitation counseling. The specific information required will depend on the purpose, goals, and domain of concern of the profession.

Which theories and empirical data are selected from the various disciplines is also dependent on the profession's purpose and goals, domain of concern, and its range of legitimate tools. The general questions asked by a profession are:

Will this information help the profession to assist others in problem identification and resolution?

Will it provide useful information for developing or refining sets of guidelines for practice?

Some people have difficulty with the idea of "selecting" theories and empirical data from various disciplines. It is seen as somehow not quite right, as a surreptitious activity. They may speak of "borrowing" theories and empirical data, as if they must be returned to their rightful place. Some of these people espouse a disciplinal orientation wherein each profession creates its own theoretical knowledge. Others simply believe theories and empirical data are owned by the discipline of their origin. However, traditionally theoretical knowledge belongs to the public and should be available for use by anyone who has the interest and ability. In any event, disciplines do not use or apply theories or empirical data. If the theories and data were not used by professions, they would only collect dust.

In a neopositivistic orientation, the information contained within the theoretical foundation is not systematically organized. Information may be grouped by discipline of origin, area of domain of concern addressed, the life cycle, or along some sort of micro-macro continuum (such as individual, family, society), among others. No one way of organizing the theoretical foundation in a neopositivistic orientation is correct. In fact, the only time much attention is given to its organization is in discussion of curriculum design for professional education. Information is not systematically organized for two reasons. First, neopositivists want to avoid any suggestion of a comprehensive theory as is found in the disciplinal orientation. The other, more important reason is that the theoretical foundation is a pool of information from which any one theoretical postulate may be taken. Each postulate is viewed as separate from all other postulates. Any systematic organization would limit this perception of the individuality of postulates. Information in a theoretical foundation eventually "gets organized" in the context of a profession's various sets of guidelines for practice.

Domain of Concern

A profession's domain of concern is comprised of those areas of human experience in which members of a profession have expertise and offer assistance to others. It is, in essence, a statement of the types of problems the profession believes it can help others to identify and resolve. A profession's domain of concern may be very broad, like nursing, or more narrow, like speech pathology.

The way a domain of concern is conceptualized reflects how a profession perceives clients and, by extension, the nature of its practice. First, the domain of concern defines what is considered a problem and what is not. In any area of human experience within the domain of concern of a profession, some behavior, states of being, status of organisms, and so forth will be viewed by the profession as problems; others will not. This goes beyond the idea of what is normal or functional versus abnormal or dysfunctional. There are sometimes potential problem areas that a profession does not perceive or attend to. For example, at one time, the rehabilitation professions totally disregarded the sexual sphere of human experience. In the phenomenological orientation, this issue is dealt with more simply—a problem is any situation the client identifies as a problem. The neopositivistic orientation demands more specificity.

Second, once categories are labelled and accepted, the phenomena in them tends to be viewed only through the lens of the categories; perception and thinking can become rigid. What is categorized may be unexamined; what is not categorized may be unseen. Thus, professions must continually study the categories within their domains of concern. Attention to this task is exemplified by the American Psychiatric Association's periodic reconceptualization of psychiatry's domain of concern as illustrated in the various editions of *Diagnostic and Statistical Manual of Mental Disorders*—I, II, III, and III-R (American Psychiatric Association, 1987).

The domain of concern of a profession has two important, although somewhat different, functions. First, it forms the nucleus for the profession's sets of guidelines for practice, which are organized around the various elements of a profession's domain of concern. Each set of guidelines provides information and precepts for dealing with one element of the domain of concern.

The second function of the domain of concern is related to communication. The nature and focus of practitioner-client interaction often are expressed primarily in terms of a profession's domain of concern; one is working with a client relative to components X and Y of the profession's domain of concern. The terminology of the domain of concern is the basis for communication among practitioner, client, those significant to the client, members of other professions, and third-party payers. This important communicative role of the domain of concern demands that a profession give attention to its specificity, clarity, and completeness.

Like a theoretical foundation, a profession's domain of concern may be organized in a number of different ways, including according to: systems (e.g., motor, sensory, cognitive), types of diagnostic categories, age groups, setting (e.g., school, industry), and primary precipitating factors. There does not seem to be any dominant or ideal pattern of organization. Each profession tends to organize its domain of concern in a way that is meaningful and useful to that profession. *The Uniform Terminology for Occupational Therapists* (Second Edition) is an example of one way of organizing a domain of concern (American Occupational Therapy Association, 1989).

Legitimate Tools

Legitimate tools are those activities, instruments, modalities, methods, techniques, and processes in which members of a profession have expertise, and which they use as the media for assisting clients (Mosey, 1986). Perhaps more than any other component of its fundamental body of knowledge, a profession holds its legitimate tools in high regard. Moreover, they come to represent or symbolize the profession both within and outside of the field—the stethoscope and medicine, for example. This may be due to the tangible qualities of many legitimate tools compared to a profession's philosophical assumptions or domain of concern.

The tools of a profession are described as "legitimate" because they are viewed as permissible for use by the profession. Their use is seen as in accordance with established tradition. In some cases, tools are literally legitimated by licensure laws. Practitioners who use tools not considered legitimate for their profession are often viewed as deviant and may be negatively sanctioned by the profession, by other professions, or by law. The legitimacy of a tool for one profession as opposed to another may cause conflict between professions, leading to the need for negotiations of some sort. This is exemplified in the conflict between physical therapists and occupational therapists over the use of physical agent modalities.

The legitimate tools of a profession change over time due to several factors: (a) a tool may be found to be ineffective, (b) one tool may be replaced by a more refined or sophisticated tool, possibly related to advances in technology, and (c) tools may be added to a profession's repertoire because of additions to its domain of concern. Changes in a profession's legitimate tools, whether deletions or additions, may be disruptive to a profession. The deletion of a tool may be experienced as a loss for some members. Additions frequently require time for understanding and mastery.

Due to the multiple meanings attached to legitimate tools, they sometimes take on a life of their own—"purposeful activities" in occupational therapy, for example. They are seen as something more than tools, somehow central to the profession. It is hard for some to see tools as "just tools," as instruments, and as means to an end. Legitimate tools have meaning and utility only in the context of a profession's sets of guidelines for practice. This does not negate the importance of studying and understanding the properties of legitimate tools or of developing skill in their use, but such knowledge and skill alone cannot serve as the basis for practice.

The tools used by professions vary widely, with some overlap between professions. However, there is one tool that seems to be common to all professions—use-of-self. Although this tool has been defined in a number of ways, in general, *use-of-self* is a preplanned (as opposed to spontaneous) personal interaction with a client, designed to assist the client in problem identification and resolution. The way the self is used varies depending upon the client, his or her situation and current needs, and the set(s) of guidelines being employed. One may, for example, be supportive, permissive, accepting, cajoling, strict, demanding, or some variation on these themes. As a tool, use-of-self may be more or less dominant in a profession's repertoire, but it is almost always there. Use-of-self should not be confused with the art of practice. The latter has a particular meaning in the neopositivistic orientation, and a meaning different from that in the phenomenological orientation. The art of practice is discussed in Chapter 5.

To summarize, in the neopositivistic orientation, each profession has a fundamental body of knowledge consisting of five categories of knowledge: philosophical assumptions, code of ethics, theoretical foundation, domain of concern, and legitimate tools. Each of these categories of knowledge are interrelated and evolve over time to meet the ever-changing needs of society. A profession's fundamental body of knowledge serves as the foundation for, supports, and reflects its applied body of knowledge.

4. Applied Body of Knowledge

A profession's applied body of knowledge is a collection of information formulated so that it serves as the basis for day-to-day problem identification and resolution with clients. More specifically, it consists of a profession's sets of guidelines for practice and evaluation procedures used for preliminary screening. An applied body of knowledge is derived from, or compatible with, the profession's fundamental body of knowledge. A profession has an applied body of knowledge because the information contained within a fundamental body of knowledge is not meant to be used directly.

Screening tools will not be discussed in any detail in this text. The focus for this chapter is the *sets of guidelines for practice*—internally consistent assemblages of information extrapolated from, or compatible with, theories or empirical data that provide direction for facilitating problem identification and fostering problem resolution in relationship to specified component(s) of a profession's domain of concern. Examples of sets of guidelines for practice are the diagnostic categories of medicine and the frames of reference of occupational therapy.

So Little Is Known

More is unknown about sets of guidelines for practice than is known. As has been previously discussed, the process of how the foundations for practice are extrapolated from theoretical information has not been adequately explained. In other words, applied Type I scientific inquiry is not well-understood. It remains recondite both because it is quite complex and because it has been little studied. A number of other factors contribute to the lack of understanding of sets of guidelines for practice.

Medicine is generally recognized as the first health profession. Unfortunately, we do not know how the structure for its sets of guidelines for practice was developed. By the time of the first written records, medicine's way of organizing information was fairly well-established, including the structural components of signs and symptoms, etiology, treatment, and so forth, but we have no idea how information came to be organized in such a fashion (Ackerknecht, 1968; Wulff et al., 1986). Moreover, we accept this received organization to such an extent that it is rarely questioned or examined, giving rise to two difficulties.

First, medicine is frequently used as a model for other health professions. Therefore, if medicine's sets of guidelines for practice are diagnostic categories, what are the sets of guidelines of the other health professions? With some exceptions, most health professions realize the structure of diagnostic categories is inappropriate for their sets of guidelines. However, other professions do look at the way medicine organizes information for practice for clues about organizing information in their own profession because it is the only structure available for study.

The second difficulty is that medicine's sets of guidelines for practice do not include a specific place for theoretical information. Although most treatment in modern medicine is based on theories and empirical data (with varying degrees of validity), theoretical information is not one of the structural components of diagnostic categories. More than likely, the lack of a structural component is due to the antiquity of diagnostic categories. When the various structural components came into being, theoretical information was not a part of medical practice. Relatively speaking, scientific medicine is a very recent phenomenon. The lack of a well-articulated, structural relationship between theoretical knowledge and practice in medicine inhibits understanding of this relationship in the other health professions.

We have recently been given an extraordinary opportunity to observe development of the content of a diagnostic category—acquired immune deficiency syndrome (AIDS). Tentatively identified in 1982, this syndrome has received much attention in the media. The struggle to understand and delineate signs and symptoms, pathology, etiology, prevention, treatment/management, and course has become a more public event than is usual for most new diagnostic categories. This is also true regarding the search for sufficient theoretical information about the HIV virus to allow for effective medical treatment, management, and, if possible, prevention. The opportunity to observe the basic and applied scientific inquiry related to AIDS may assist us in gaining better understanding of how sets of guidelines for practice in general are developed, refined, and assessed. Examples from this process will be used occasionally in the text.

Four additional factors, unrelated to medicine, seem to contribute to the lack of understanding of sets of guidelines for practice. One is that developing sets of guidelines for practice is a covert activity in many professions. Sets of guidelines tend to be formed in a piecemeal manner with contributions from many people and with little understanding of what is being formed or the processes involved. Theoretically based sets of guidelines for practice gradually emerge, but we are not sure how.

Furthermore, sets of guidelines for practice are often employed without practitioners' full understanding of their use. When questioned, a practitioner usually is able to describe how a particular problem would be identified and resolved. And, in retrospect, many are able to describe a theoretical basis for their past actions. However, theory is often not seen as a part of problem identification and resolution; rather, it is viewed as information separate from practice.

The third factor is related to the traditional structure of professional education—that is, the basic sciences followed by "clinical courses." This structure, recommended by Flexner in his seminal report on medical education in 1910, has been followed by most of the health professions. Such a structure fosters—if not encourages—a split between theoretical knowledge and practice (Thorne, 1973). Theoretical information is taught isolated from the sets of guidelines for the practice that it supports. Clinical courses frequently present sets of guidelines for practice disconnected from the theoretical information fundamental to them, making the guidelines only a series of techniques. Students are left to make the connection between theoretical information and practice unaided by instruction. On the other hand, when theoretical information is mentioned in clinical courses, it may be in such a general manner that specific postulates supporting a given set of guidelines for practice are not identified. As a result of such an education, practitioners tend to compartmentalize their learning, separating theoretical knowledge from problem identification and resolution.

The last factor inhibiting understanding of sets of guidelines for practice is the absence of designated "middle persons" (Van Melsen, 1961). Traditionally, professions have left the development of sets of guidelines to anyone who expresses an interest. While professions speak of the roles of practitioner, educator, and administrator, they hardly acknowledge the importance of applied scientists—the middle persons. In most health professions, it is unclear who these applied scientists are, how they fit into the typically designated professional roles, and how they should be educated. It is often assumed that "everyone should do a little research" or, with hope more than anything else, that educators are the applied scientists of professions.

Recently, professions have become more concerned about scientific inquiry, offering courses at the professional and postprofessional levels. However, courses tend to focus on research design rather than the broader perspective of scientific inquiry. Kerlinger (1960) was concerned about this matter 30 years ago; unfortunately there seems to have been little change since then. When courses do focus on scientific inquiry, the majority of attention is usually given to basic inquiry as opposed to applied. As a result, practitioners tend to be ill-prepared for the task of developing, refining, and assessing the adequacy of sets of guidelines for practice.

By What Name Should We Call Them?

The lack of understanding regarding sets of guidelines for practice is perhaps best exemplified by the absence of either a specific name for them in most professions or a generic term across all professions. A review of the literature of the health professions and the philosophy of science and technology provided the following labels for what has been referred to here as sets of guidelines for practice: theory (Henderson,

1988), practice theory or theory of practice (Fitzpatrick & Whall, 1983), prescriptive theory (Beckstrand, 1986; Yerxa, 1981), model of practice (Llorens & Gillette, 1985), linking structure (Mosey, 1981, 1986), ground rules (Bunge, 1983), modus operandi (Feibleman, 1983), and guidelines for action (Van Melsen, 1961). The ideas to which each of these labels was attached were poorly defined, but all seemed to refer to either "that which serves as the immediate basis for practice" or "the end product of applied scientific inquiry." All referred to the transformation of theoretical knowledge into a form that allowed it to be used in practice.

The rationale for the name, *sets of guidelines for practice*, follows:

The term "theory" was rejected for two reasons. First, theories are very different entities than sets of guidelines for practice. Theories and sets of guidelines are dissimilar relative to origin, structure, content, and function, as well as in the way they are developed, refined, and evaluated. Although sets of guidelines are based on theories, they are not theories. Second, sets of guidelines for practice never evolve into theories. The complex relationship between theoretical information and sets of guidelines for practice, and between basic and applied scientific inquiry was suggested in Chapter 1 and will be discussed further in Chapter 9. Naming sets of guidelines for practice "theory"—with or without a modifying term—is inappropriate, considered poor scholarship, and confusing.

The term "prescriptive" is frequently used in the literature to describe sets of guidelines for practice. "Prescriptive" refers to a course of action to be taken and, in that sense, is a characteristic of sets of guidelines for practice. On the other hand, prescriptive also denotes rules laid down by others to be followed without variation. Sets of guidelines for practice are not rules in this sense but, rather, provide suggested ways of proceeding in regards to problem identification and resolution. Their application requires judgment on the part of the practitioner and modification, within limits, to meet the needs of a particular client. Sets of guidelines suggest a course of action, but are not rules to be blindly followed.

The term "model" has many meanings. Use of the term by the health professions, scientists, and philosophers has become so extensive and variable that it seems to have lost any specific meaning. Wartofsky (1979) has written an informative and well-titled chapter, "The Model Muddle." Because of its overuse and lack of precise meaning, "model" did not seem an appropriate term for sets of guidelines for practice.

"Linking structure" is another term used as a label for sets of guidelines for practice. The advantage of this term, which has been used by the author in the past, is its designation of an important function of sets of guidelines—linking theoretical knowledge to practice. The disadvantage is that it implies only that function. In other words, it does not indicate the major function of sets of guidelines for practice, which is their use in problem identification and resolution with clients.

"Ground rules," sometimes used by philosophers of technology, seemed a bit vague. "Modus operandi," a method of operating or working, also seemed too vague. Its association with the "M.O." of suspected perpetrators on crime shows on television also contributed to the author's feeling that it was not an appropriate label.

Van Melsen (1961) used the term "guidelines for action." With the addition of the word, "set," this term was selected as the higher order concept referring to the end products of applied Type I scientific inquiry, which result in a foundation for making (sets of technological guidelines) and for doing (sets of guidelines for practice). "Guidelines" seemed appropriate because of its meaning of a suggested course of action—"to assist (a person) to travel through or reach a destination" in an area of uncertainty and often-changing terrain (Flexner & Hauck, 1987). The modifier "set" was added to indicate that a collection of related guidelines are used as the basis for identifying and resolving specific problems. Finally, "practice" was chosen as a subelement of "action" because it is the term used by members of the health professions to denote their particular kind of action.

Not only do many professions working within a neopositivistic orientation not have a name for their sets of guidelines for practice, but they also have difficulty in describing the structure and required content of their bases for practice. This is not to say these professions are unconcerned about their applied body of knowledge. They engage in considerable applied scientific inquiry directed towards developing and refining means for problem identification and resolution relating to their domain of concern. The entities created have the characteristics of sets of guidelines for practice suitable for that profession. The lack of a name—and the corresponding lack of awareness of what is being created—may be due to a feeling of such intuitive familiarity with practice that labelling and defining specifications of required structure and content do not seem necessary.

Sets of Guidelines for Practice

The following section provides an overview of sets of guidelines for practice. Attention is given to (a) functions, (b) structure, (c) relationship of content to a fundamental body of knowledge, and (d) some relevant issues related to adequacy.[1]

Functions

Sets of guidelines for practice fulfill a variety of functions for professions. First, they integrate theoretical information and practice by linking problems encountered in practice with theoretical knowledge. Practice founded on theoretical information is generally believed to lead to more effective problem identification and resolution than practice based on the "particular solutions" of the traditional epistemological orientation.

Second, the structure of sets of guidelines for practice provides the framework for analyzing, selecting, and synthesizing theoretical information. It specifies required content, thereby assisting in (a) identifying potentially appropriate theories and empirical data, (b) determining what particular postulates are useful, and (c) extrapolating from these postulates in such a way that they can be used to meet the practical goals of a profession. Sets of guidelines can be viewed as a transitional structure, assisting in the change of theoretical information to information useful in practice.

Third, sets of guidelines for practice are the means whereby a profession organizes its collection of ap-

[1]Much of the information presented in this section is drawn from the work of Beckstrand (1986), Bunge (1983), Fleming, Johnson, Marina, Spergel, and Townson (1987), Glaser (1976), Hardy (1973), Hilgard and Bower (1974), J. K. Larsen (1981), and Mosey (1981, 1986).

plied knowledge. Rather than being left as a haphazard jumble of information, applied knowledge is grouped and arranged in a systematic manner around the elements of the profession's domain of concern. Adequate organization of an applied body of knowledge allows practitioners to select necessary information quickly and accurately. A well-organized applied body of knowledge is analogous to one's dresser drawers—if they are organized in some sort of known manner, there is no need to search through every drawer to find two matching socks.

Related to their function of organizing applied knowledge, sets of guidelines for practice strongly influence the way practitioners think. They influence how information is processed, how problems are viewed, and how theoretical information is considered. Members of a profession are so unaware of how they process information that they give it little attention. For example, physicians think like physicians; they think in terms of diagnostic categories in the clinical setting, when reading theoretical and professional literature, and, perhaps, while involved in leisure activities. Individuals who have had experience working with practitioners from many different professions may at one time or another have said, "you think like a social worker," or "...like a recreational therapist." Occasionally this may be said in exasperation, but mostly it is said to indicate that one knows the perspective of the other practitioner—how he or she is processing information.

The fifth and most obvious function of sets of guidelines is their use in practice. They provide the information needed to make judgments about what assessment procedures may be useful and which intervention strategies are most likely to be successful. They serve as the basis of day-to-day clinical reasoning, decision making, and action.

Paradoxically, the final function of sets of guidelines is that they clearly indicate what a profession does *not* know. They identify the gaps in a profession's theoretical and applied knowledge. Examination of a profession's sets of guidelines for practice allows the profession to determine:

1. What sets of guidelines are based on theories and empirical data of questionable validity or

Applied Scientific Inquiry in the Health Professions

are, in fact, atheoretical.

2. The extent to which strategies for problem identification and resolution are stated in a precise
manner.

3. The adequacy of the various sets of guidelines—in terms of safety, effectiveness, efficiency, and acceptability to clients.

4. Those aspects of the profession's domain of concern for which there are no sets of guidelines.

5. What additional theoretical information is
needed by the profession.

It is only through honest assessment of sets of
guidelines for practice that professions are able to
identify the appropriate focus of their applied scientific inquiry. A clear focus gives inquiry direction and
meaning so that the same problems are not "researched
to death," but, rather, new and sometimes more difficult areas are examined.

Structure   "Structure" refers to the parts of sets of guidelines for
practice and how these parts are arranged. The struc-
ture of sets of guidelines varies from profession to
profession, with no one structure able to be applied to
all on the basis of logic or practicality. A structure is
developed and accepted because it has specific relevance to a given profession. It is designed to meet a
profession's needs and is used because it meets those
needs. However, sets of guidelines of different professions may have analogous parts. For instance, the
structure for sets of guidelines for medicine is (a) signs
and symptoms, (b) pathology, (c) etiology, (d) prevention, (e) treatment/management, (f) course, and (g)
sequelae. In contrast, the structure of occupational
therapy's sets of guidelines is (a) theoretical base, (b)
function/dysfunction continua, (c) behaviors and
physical signs indicative of function and dysfunction,
and (d) postulates regarding change. The parts of each
of these sets of guidelines are very different, but com-
parisons can be made. Signs and symptoms are in
some way similar to behaviors and physical signs
indicative of function and dysfunction; treatment/
management, in the sense of alleviating a problem, is
similar to postulates regarding change. Although there
are analogous parts in the structures of some set of
guidelines for practice, care must be taken to remember that these are only analogies, not equivalencies.

The degree of difference and similarity between the sets of guidelines for practice of the various health professions is probably related to the types of problems they deal with. For instance, the sets of guidelines of medicine and of occupational therapy are quite dissimilar because medicine is primarily concerned with the treatment of disease whereas occupational therapy is primarily concerned with habilitation/rehabilitation. The only major meeting point is in the area of sequelae. If physical therapy had a specifically stated structure for its sets of guidelines, it would probably be more similar to occupational therapy than to medicine, as it also is concerned primarily with habilitation/rehabilitation.

The sequence of practice, the way in which members of a profession go about the process of problem identification and proceed through to problem resolution, is at least partially reflected in the structure of the profession's sets of guidelines for practice. By identifying the types of information needed, the various parts that will eventually make up the structure of the profession's set of guidelines begin to emerge. Subsequently, the structure is refined so as to be of particular relevance to the profession.

Finally, with the exception of medicine, sets of guidelines for practice of health professions are likely to need a structure that includes a category for theoretical information basic to the set of guidelines. Such a category allows for easy recognition of the theoretical foundation (or lack thereof) for a given set of guidelines. It also assists the profession in identifying the requisite theoretical information needed to support new sets of guidelines for practice.

Relationship of Content to a Fundamental Body of Knowledge

The content of a profession's fundamental body of knowledge is reflected in the collective content of its sets of guidelines for practice. The philosophical assumptions of a profession regarding the individual, the environment, and the profession's goals provide broad parameters for what is and is not included in the profession's sets of guidelines for practice. A profession's code of ethics establishes boundaries relative to the methods and strategies of evaluation and intervention that are morally permissible.

The relationship between the theoretical foundation of a profession and the theoretical content of its sets of guidelines for practice is ideally one of agreement. The theories and empirical data included in a profession's sets of guidelines for practice constitute the theoretical foundation of the profession. As a profession adds, refines, and deletes sets of guidelines, so too is the content of its theoretical foundation altered. If a profession only used the current content of its theoretical foundation, there would be minimal change or advancement in its sets of guidelines for practice. Typically, newly developed sets of guidelines for practice are not based on information that is part of a profession's existing theoretical foundation. When such a set of guidelines is demonstrated to be adequate, or at least believed to be adequate, the theoretical information basic to the new set of guidelines is added to the profession's theoretical foundation. This can be seen, for example, in the development by several health professions of sets of guidelines related to adjustment problems of the elderly. Theoretical information regarding the normal aging process and its attendant typical life situations were added to the theoretical foundation of these professions.

However, the process may not be that simple. A new set of guidelines for practice may be rejected for a period of time because the supporting theories or empirical data are not accepted by the profession. For example, the theory of pathogenic microorganisms was not accepted by surgeons; thus, the use of sterile techniques was considered to be unnecessary and odd. Another example is the difficulty that occupational therapists had in accepting sets of guidelines for practice based in part on learning theories. Indeed, to this day some educational programs give little instruction in learning theories, and some occupational therapists avoid recognizing their importance to the profession. Difficulty in accepting new sets of guidelines for practice is often due to factors other than the perceived validity of the underlying theoretical knowledge. In the above examples, it is thought that the use of sterile techniques may have offended the macho image of surgeons (Ackerknecht, 1968). For occupational therapists, it may be the association of learning theories with being "craft teachers."

The elements of a profession's domain of concern serve as the nucleus of its sets of guidelines, with each set of guidelines addressing one element. Thus, the domain of concern often serves as a boundary for permissible sets of guidelines. The sets of guidelines of a profession concerned with ameliorating the psychosocial effects of illness or disability will have different content than those of a profession concerned with maintaining adequate nutrition during a disease process.

Occasionally, sets of guidelines for practice may be developed that are outside of, or only tangentially related to, a profession's domain of concern. This occurs when the profession moves into new areas of human experience. An extreme example of this process can be seen in the medical specialty of radiology (Bucher & Strauss, 1961). Initially concerned primarily with diagnoses, radiology moved into the treatment of a variety of disease conditions. Because this was a major departure from the specialty's original domain of concern, multiple new sets of guidelines needed to be developed, and, consequently, the nature of this medical specialty changed dramatically.

While the example of radiology is unusual, as society identifies new needs, individuals move outside of their profession's domain of concern in an attempt to meet these needs. If the newly developed sets of guidelines for practice are accepted by the profession, the area of human experience central to the set of guidelines becomes an element of the profession's domain of concern. On the other hand, the profession may reject the set of guidelines and, therefore, the area of human experience addressed therein. Although many factors may influence rejection, the major factor is likely to be the profession's philosophical assumptions. The area of human experience may be seen as too far removed from what the profession sees as its purpose and goals.

The legitimate tools of a profession shape the content of its sets of guidelines for practice in a number of ways. First, selected theories and empirical data must ultimately provide information about how these tools are to be used. Legitimate tools usually have a wide potential for use—sometimes more than the profession is aware of—but they also have invariant characteristics and limits, and they can be stretched only so far. For example, creative activities in the plastic arts— painting, sculpting, drawing, construction—are some of the legitimate tools of art therapy. The theoretical information that serves as the basis for sets of guidelines for practice for this profession must be compatible with the possible uses of these tools. Thus, some theoretical information would not be suitable. Extrapolation from this information would logically require use of tools not considered legitimate by art therapists. For example, theoretical information about the therapeutic properties of heat would not be part of the theoretical foundation of art therapy. Such information supports the use of physical agent modalities, such as hot packs and ultrasound, tools that are not use by art therapists.

Second, the legitimate tools of a profession establish limits with regard to the methods used for problem identification. A physical therapist, for example, would use far different evaluation strategies to identify a client's degree of motivation than a psychologist would use. Third, legitimate tools shape that part of sets of guidelines for practice that deals with problem resolution. Sets of guidelines give direction for selecting appropriate tools and for how these tools are to be used.

Finally, the addition of new legitimate tools is likely to influence a profession's sets of guidelines for practice. The addition of an entirely new tool is rare, but tools are often refined or expanded in some way. One example of change due to expansion is the development of antibiotics. Therapeutic drugs in various forms have been used by medicine for centuries, but antibiotics were a whole different class of drugs. New treatment possibilities opened up; medicine was able to rewrite many of its sets of guidelines for practice.

Some Issues Related to Adequacy

This section deals with some general issues related to sets of guidelines for practice, many of them concerned with adequacy in a broad sense. Specific issues related to adequacy and assessment are discussed in Chapter 10. The issues discussed are: (a) what determines the number of sets of guidelines in a profession, (b) along what dimensions do sets vary, (c) incompatibility among sets of guidelines, and (d) interprofessional similarity of sets of guidelines.

The number of sets of guidelines included in a profession's applied body of knowledge appears to depend on two factors. One, previously mentioned, is the breadth of a profession's domain of concern. The other factor seems to be the profession's extent of experience with the neopositivistic orientation. Some professions in transition from a traditional to a neopositivistic orientation may still use many particular solutions as the basis for practice. Professions moving from a disciplinal to a neopositivistic orientation may not have developed sets of guidelines for many elements of their domain of concern.

The sets of guidelines for practice of any profession tend to vary along several dimensions. One dimension is the extent to which sets of guidelines are based on valid theories and empirical data. All professions attempt to use the most valid theoretical information currently available, but the information in some areas of human experience is far more valid than in others. We know more, for example, about the musculoskeletal system than the central nervous system. Some theories are based more on speculation—or even wishful thinking—than on sound research findings. Less-than-valid theoretical information is used because there is simply nothing else available. A profession is judged according to whether or not it uses the most valid theoretical information currently available as the foundation for its sets of guidelines for practice. It is considered acceptable to use a theory of questionable validity when it is the only theory available. It is not acceptable to use such a theory when an appropriate theory with a higher degree of validity exists.

Another dimension along which sets of guidelines vary is their degree of completeness. On close inspection, some sets of guidelines for practice may be only tentatively or tangentially based on theoretical knowledge. Others may not provide sufficient information regarding problem identification. Still others may have minimal guidelines relative to problem resolution. A third dimension is degree of specificity both in relationship to structure and to content. Some professions seem to be more comfortable with sets of guidelines that are loosely structured and provide very general direction for practice, while others prefer more highly structured sets of guidelines and more specific directions for problem identification and resolution. Another dimension is the extent to which the adequacy of various sets of guidelines for practice have been assessed. In most professions, some sets of guidelines have been assessed in considerable detail, while others have not. The recency of the development of a set of guidelines is a contributing factor, of course. A final dimension is degree of effectiveness, which is related to assessment of adequacy. The probability of effectiveness in problem resolution for some sets of guidelines is often quite high, while for others rather low. Sets of guidelines with a low probability of effectiveness usually continue to be used only because there is simply no better set of guidelines available. They should be used only when practitioner and client are fully aware of their low probability of success.

The third issue in considering the collection of a profession's sets of guidelines for practice is compatibility. Given essentially the same information, each of two sets of guidelines may identify and describe a problem in a different manner. For example, using one set of guidelines, a client's difficulties in functioning may be identified as primarily intrapsychic in nature. Using another set of guidelines, the problem may be seen as lack of adequate skills to manage everyday demands of the environment. Of course, the strategies suggested for problem resolution would also be different in these two sets of guidelines for practice.

Sets of guidelines for practice may be compatible with regard to problem identification but not in terms of strategies for problem resolution. In other words, there may be general agreement about the nature of the problem but not about the course of action that should be taken to deal with the problem. For instance, the methods for identifying breast cancer are uncontroversial; however, there are many competing ideas about which treatments are best.

Although the incompatibility of sets of guidelines for practice within a profession is often troublesome, such a situation may force the profession to give more attention to the inquiry needed to refine and assess the adequacy of the sets of guidelines in question. Because assessment is often a lengthy process, the incompatible sets of guidelines remain part of the profession's applied body of knowledge in the interim. Lacking sound scientific data, practitioners select from competing sets of guidelines based on their clinical experience, judgment, and personal preference.

The final issue to be noted is interprofessional

similarity of sets of guidelines for practice. At times, similarities are more apparent than real. Since some theories and empirical data are shared by several professions, sets of guidelines of these professions must be based, at least in part, on the same theoretical information. However, this does not mean the subsequent sets of guidelines will be the same because a profession's *entire* fundamental body of knowledge shapes its sets of guidelines. In illustration, occupational therapy and early childhood special education share various theories that collectively stress that engaging in "doing" facilitates the acquisition of knowledge and skills. They also share a common legitimate tool—play activities. However, the sets of guidelines of the two professions are quite different, due to differences in their domains of concern, purposes, and goals. Occupational therapists use play activities primarily to remediate sequelae of illnesses, injuries, or genetic aberrations; special education teachers use them primarily to facilitate academic learning.

On the other hand, there are professions that do have some sets of guidelines for practice in common— particularly those professions that are closely related in some area. For example, clinical psychology and social work, in their shared concern with problems in adjustment, have similar sets of guidelines relative to psychotherapy and counseling. The differences between the professions' applied bodies of knowledge are generally more distinct than between their fundamental bodies of knowledge. Nevertheless, most professions have at least a few sets of guidelines for practice in common with another profession.

An Example of a Set of Guidelines for Practice: Frame of Reference

Two different sets of guidelines for practice, diagnostic categories and frames of reference, have been mentioned repeatedly in this text. Diagnostic categories are likely to be familiar to the reader from either direct use, working closely with physicians, or life experience. In order to give the reader further understanding of sets of guidelines for practice, the structure and content of frames of reference are briefly outlined (Mosey 1981, 1986). There are four parts to a frame of reference:

Theoretical Base

The theoretical base of a frame of reference is an integrated system of postulates that describes an element of the profession's domain of concern, components of that element (if any), and environmental factors that positively influence the element addressed. It provides information fundamental (a) to identifying a state of function or dysfunction and (b) to enhancing function and/or modifying dysfunction in the specified area. The term "theoretical base" is used to indicate that this part of a frame of reference is made up of theoretical information and is the matrix from which all other parts of the frame of reference are derived.

To be more specific, the theoretical base defines and describes the nature of the area of human experience to which the frame of reference is addressed and the subdivisions of that area, if appropriate. For example, in a frame of reference concerned with memory, memory may be conceived of as a singular entity or as an entity best described as being made up of various components of memory, such as short-term, long-term, recent, and remote. Second, the theoretical base provides general information about behavior and physical signs typical of an individual who has problems in the area addressed. Third, postulates describing environmental factors—both human and nonhuman—that positively influence the area addressed are delineated. Environmental factors are of particular importance in occupational therapy because intervention involves designing environments that enhance function.

The theoretical base of a frame of reference may be formulated out of one theory, or postulates may be drawn from several theories or empirical data. The latter is most often the case. Some dynamic postulates are always included in the theoretical base.

Function–Dysfunction
Continua

The element or its components being addressed in the frame of reference form the function–dysfunction continua. There may be one continuum, the area addressed in the frame of reference, or several continua, the components of the area. If, for example, memory was conceived of as a singular entity, there would be one continuum. If memory was described as having various components, there would be four continua: short-term memory, long-term memory, and so forth. Most frames of reference have more than one continuum because (a) the areas addressed in frames of reference tend to be complex, and (b) dividing an area into components often allows for more refined problem identification and resolution. Collectively, the continua are the possible problem areas investigated and resolved through use of the frame of reference.

The term "continuum" is used to emphasize the lack of a strict line of demarcation between what is considered functional and what is considered dysfunctional. Function and dysfunction are viewed as relative to age, cultural group membership, life style, present life circumstances, and any other pertinent factors.

Behaviors and Physical Signs Indicative of Function and Dysfunction

Behaviors and physical signs that indicate function and dysfunction are actions, verbal statements, and biological data specific to each continuum that are used as the basis for problem identification with a client. By referring to these indicators, the client and practitioner determine whether a problem exists and, if so, what the specific nature of that problem is. For instance, some of the behavioral indicators of short-term-memory dysfunction might be the inability to remember what one ate for breakfast, what day it is, or what one did yesterday.

Behaviors and physical signs indicative of function and dysfunction are also the framework used for designing evaluation procedures such as interviews, physical examinations, and tests designed to observe performance in specific areas. Finally, these indicators are used, when appropriate, as the starting point for developing standardized evaluation procedures.

Postulates Regarding Change

Postulates regarding change are specific statements or precepts that describe the characteristics, quality, quantity, and sequence of interaction with the human and nonhuman environment that, according to the theoretical base, will enhance function or decrease dysfunction in the area addressed in the frame of reference. They are used to design environments for problem resolution. Within the limits imposed by the frame of reference, such environments are designed to take into consideration the needs, values, beliefs, interests, and current life situation of the client.

A frame of reference either begins or ends with information about the boundaries of the frame of reference. This usually includes a description of the population for which the frame of reference is considered suitable in terms of age, functional levels, and, if appropriate, specific diagnoses. Contraindications are also specified.

Applied Scientific Inquiry in the Health Professions

It should be remembered that a frame of reference is only one type of set of guidelines for practice. Frames of reference are not suitable for medicine, just as diagnostic categories are not suitable for occupational therapy. Each profession, then, has a type of sets of guidelines to meet its own particular practice needs.

Practice and Technology

The purpose of this section is to sort out the similarities, differences, and relationships between sets of guidelines for practice and sets of technological guidelines (Galdston, 1981; Goldstein, 1988; Grove, 1989; Weissman, 1991; Wulff, Pedersen, & Rosenberg, 1986). The technology of concern here involves the fabrication of objects used for maintaining or restoring health or enhancing the quality of life of those with impaired health. These physical objects—medication, instruments, machines, apparatus, equipment, appliances, prostheses, braces, splints, and the like—are referred to as technological products.

Technology—in the form of preparation of herbs and devices to deal with illness—has been a part of medicine since its inception. As other health professions evolved, some have made considerable use of technological products, while others have not. Today, the majority of health professions make use of technology in one way or another. Indeed, practitioners of some professions may feel overwhelmed by the number of technological products available for their use.

Several sequential processes are involved in formulating theoretically based technological products and their incorporation into sets of guidelines for practice. These are outlined in the center of Figure 3.

To briefly summarize the processes, applied Type I scientific inquiry, which is typically instigated by a problem that is primarily technological in nature, is used to develop a set of technological guidelines. This set of guidelines in turn is used as the blueprint, either literally or figuratively, for fabricating a technological product. Using applied Type II inquiry, the product is first tested in the laboratory or field for such qualities as safety, reliability, and effectiveness. Following any necessary refinement, the product is subjected to *clinical* testing and, if necessary, further refined and tested. Both laboratory/field and clinical testing address such questions as how, when, what amount of, with whom, and under what circumstances the product should be used or has potential for use.

After a technological product is demonstrated to be safe, reliable, and effective relative to specified criteria, it may be incorporated into a set of guidelines for practice. Applied Type I inquiry is again used. The product may become part of a previously formulated sets of guidelines. On the other hand, if the product is revolutionary, a new set of guidelines for practice may be formulated. The former is illustrated in the development of a more effective drug for a clearly defined pathological process. An example of the latter is the use of new technological products in the care of low birth weight infants. Finally, Applied Type II inquiry is used to assess the adequacy of the altered or new set of guidelines for practice.

The extent to which a given health profession is involved in developing sets of technological guidelines as opposed to just using technological products varies. Four categories of professions are described below; a particular profession may fall somewhere between two categories.

Technology as Primary Focus

Professions within this category are primarily concerned with fabricating health-related products and formulating sets of technological guidelines for them. Examples of such professions include bioengineering and that aspect of pharmacy concerned with developing drugs and related medicinal substances. Following the sequence outlined in Figure 3, professions with technology as a primary focus are usually responsible for the process through the laboratory or field testing of the product (indicated on the top half of Figure 3). The clinical testing phase almost always takes place in partnership with practitioners who are likely to be consumers of the product in question. Because professions with technology as a primary focus are usually not involved in direct client care, their applied bodies of knowledge consist of sets of technological guidelines, not sets of guidelines for practice.

Consumers of Technological Products

Professions that are consumers of technological products are primarily concerned with the use of technological products and sometimes with laboratory/field testing (bottom half of Figure 3). A few examples of consumer professions are medicine, nursing, and

Figure 3. The role of professions in the process of developing health-related technological products and the inclusion of these products in sets of guidelines for practice.

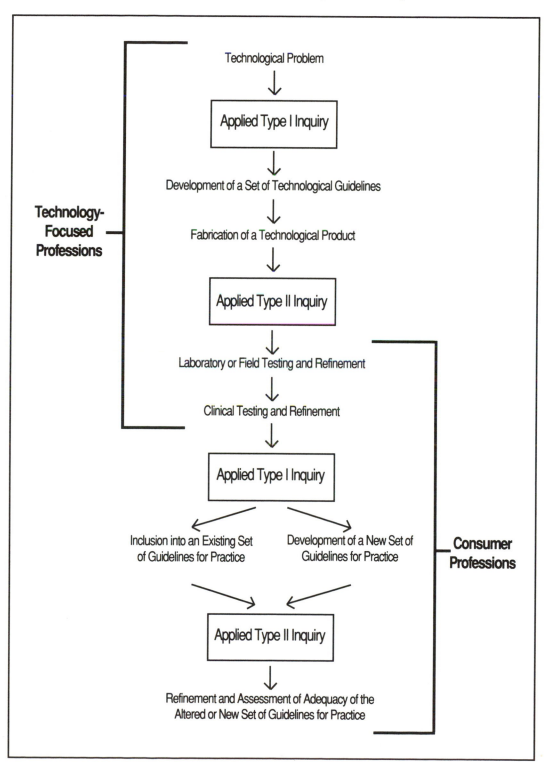

physical therapy. The applied bodies of knowledge of consumer professions rarely, if ever, include sets of technological guidelines for that is not their primary focus. Rather, they are concerned with the clinical assessment of technological products and, when satisfied with the assessment results, incorporating these products into sets of guidelines for practice.

Members of consumer professions may request development of technological products and assist in outlining specific needs. However, they usually are not involved in the applied Type I inquiry necessary for formulating sets of technological guidelines or in product fabrication. Consumer professions are concerned with the use of technological products within the broader process of assisting clients in problem identification and resolution.

Mixed Consumer and Technological Focus

The applied body of knowledge of mixed consumer/technological focused professions includes both sets of technological guidelines and sets of guidelines for practice, with the latter usually being predominant. Two examples of professions in this category are dentistry and occupational therapy. Some aspects of occupational therapy involve designing and fabricating various types of equipment to facilitate independent functioning. To do this, occupational therapists need to develop, refine, and assess sets of technological guidelines. In mixed professions when a technological product is found to be safe, reliable, and effective, the set of technological guidelines becomes part of the profession's applied body of knowledge. The product itself is incorporated into one or more sets of guidelines for practice. In occupational therapy, splinting is frequently incoporated into the sets of guidelines for practice for various hand injuries. The use of splints, however, is usually only one element of the total problem resolution regimen suggested by the sets of guidelines.

Minimal Use of Technological Products

Some professions, like social work and rehabilitation counseling, do not use, or make minimal use of, technological products in directly assisting clients. This is not to imply that members of these professions are not consumers of technological products outside of clinical activities; they frequently make use of such products in scientific inquiry, record keeping, and communication.

In conclusion, it is important to note the difference between sets of technological guidelines and sets of guidelines for practice. Sets of technological guidelines are concerned with the fabrication of technological products. Although sets of guidelines for practice may include the use of technological products, their emphasis is on providing direction for problem identification and resolution with clients. Technological products may facilitate this process.

5. Practice

The third level of organization in a neopositivistic orientation is practice, which includes information basic to skilled and ethical use of a profession's applied body of knowledge for the purpose of collaborative problem identification and resolution with clients. A profession's fundamental body of knowledge remains in the background in the immediacy of practice, except for philosophical assumptions and a code of ethics that always permeate practice.

Three dimensions of practice are described: (a) aspects and sequence of practice, (b) use of an applied body of knowledge, and (c) clinical reasoning and decision making. This is followed by discussion of some problem areas related to the use of an applied body of knowledge. Finally, the art of practice from the neopositivistic perspective is outlined.

Three Dimensions of Practice

Practice involves multiple processes and is perhaps best viewed as three-dimensional. Because the dimensions of practice described here are interrelated and overlapping, each dimension can be understood only in the context of the other two.

Aspects and Sequence of Practice

Aspects of practice are those activities and patterns of interaction that constitute the process of practice. Collectively, they describe the sequence of events from the beginning of problem identification through problem resolution and termination. This is an ideal definition; at times the problem cannot be identified or, if identified, it cannot be resolved. Aspects of practice tend to be quite similar for all health professions; however, there are variations and differences in terminology. Aspects of practice are identified here as:

1. Initial assessment (screening and formal assessment).

2. Intervention.

3. Continuing assessment (concurrent with intervention).

4. Termination.

5. Communication/documentation (throughout the process).

Initial assessment is a collaborative process between practitioner and client directed toward identifying problem areas. By extension, it also involves identifying areas where there are no problems. Initial assessment is often divided into two phases, screening and formal assessment. Screening involves ascertaining probable problem areas. The resulting findings serve as the basis for selecting sets of guidelines for practice likely to be useful in formal assessment. The purpose of formal assessment is to arrive at a more definitive statement about the nature of the client's problem or problems.

Intervention based on sets of guidelines for practice is the process of assisting a client in problem resolution. It involves goal setting, a plan or regimen of some sort, and implementation. Intervention may be viewed as a unitary process or as subdivided into various types of interventions, such as prevention, treatment, maintenance, management, and so forth. Continuing assessment is concomitant with intervention and involves evaluation of progress toward problem resolution. Termination is the process of bringing intervention to a satisfactory end. Ideally, it is synonymous with problem resolution, but of course this is not always the case.

Communication and documentation are ongoing processes, beginning with screening and continuing through termination. Communication refers to the sharing of information among practitioner, client, those significant to the client, other team members, and appropriate administrative personnel. Documentation, a more formal means of communication, is a written, ongoing record of the assessment, intervention, and termination process.

Use of an Applied Body of Knowledge

In essence, use of an applied body of knowledge is the application of selected sets of guidelines for practice with a client. After screening, one or more sets of guidelines for practice are selected as the basis for

Applied Scientific Inquiry in the Health Professions

initial formal assessment. Once problem areas are identified, appropriate sets of guidelines for practice are
used alone, in combination, or sequentially as the
basis for problem resolution. The process is not always that clear cut, however. Initially and often for
some period of time, there is movement by the practitioner back and forth between the applied body of
knowledge and work with a client. A set of guidelines
for practice may be selected, used, and found to be
appropriate for problem identification and/or effective in problem resolution with a client in a relatively
short period of time. On the other hand, some sets of
guidelines may prove to be inappropriate or ineffective for the client. One set of guidelines may be discarded, other sets of guidelines selected, another tentatively used, and so forth. This process continues
until suitable sets of guidelines for practice are found
for problem identification and resolution with the client.

In the neopositivistic orientation, assistance offered to clients is individualized. This is inherent in
the term, "guidelines," with its meaning of "suggested
ways of doing." Sets of guidelines for practice are not
rules or recipes. Within the boundaries of a given set
a guidelines, assistance is offered to a client taking into
consideration his or her perceptions; life situation;
cultural background; age; preferences; and physical,
cognitive, and emotional assets and limitations. Indi-
vidualization of practice—within guidelines derived
from theoretical knowledge—is an important characteristic of the neopositivistic orientation. This indi-
vidualization of problem identification and resolution
should not be confused with the unique-case theory of
the phenomenological orientation. In the latter, there
are no guidelines derived from theoretical information; no guidelines of any kind are used. Although
assessment and intervention are individualized as
much as possible in the neopositivistic orientation, it is
always done within the boundaries of a given set of
guidelines for practice.

Clinical Reasoning and Decision Making

The overarching intellectual processes that occur during practice—whereby conclusions are arrived at regarding a client's problem areas and the best course of
action to take for problem resolution—are referred to
as clinical reasoning and decision making. Often there
are no right answers, just multiple options; delibera-

tion and judgment are required (Dowie & Elstein, 1988; Eddy & Clanton, 1982; Lusted, 1968; Pellegrino, 1979; J. C. Rogers, 1983).

Although they have been studied fairly extensively, there is still little understanding of the mental processes involved in clinical reasoning and decision making. Most studies have used observation of the process by nonparticipants and introspection (reporting on the process in retrospect) and verbalization by participants engaged in the process. There are limitations to each of these research designs (Eddy & Clanton, 1982). Thus, until other designs are developed, important aspects of these processes will probably remain inaccessible.

From what is known, it appears that sound clinical reasoning and decision making are dependent on:

1. A store of organized professional knowledge.

2. A reasoning process to apply that knowledge.

3. The integration of a variety of information regarding the client's condition and situation with an extensive store of professional knowledge.

4. Long-term experience in engaging in the involved processes (Kassirer, Kuipers, & Gorry, 1982).

The most generally accepted idea about clinical reasoning and decision making is that they involve hypothetical-deductive reasoning—that is, generating and testing a series of hypotheses (Eddy & Clanton, 1982). Hypothetical-deductive reasoning first involves formulating an hypothesis from whatever initial data are available. Based on that hypothesis additional data are gathered. The hypothesis is tested against the new data. If the hypothesis is not supported by the new data or provides only a partial explanation for the data, another hypothesis is formed, more data are gathered, and the process continues.

In the process of clinical reasoning, practitioners draw upon the presenting situation of the client, the sets of guidelines for practice of their profession, past experience, and any new information they can garner about the client. They search for the "right fit" between the available data about the client and information contained within sets of guidelines for practice. The process continues until practitioner and client are able to arrive at some conclusion about the nature of the client's problem and the course of action to be taken in problem resolution.

Clinical reasoning and decision making takes place in the context of three major questions:

1. What is the client's current status?
2. What can be done?
3. What will be done?

These are questions involving knowledge as well as values and ethical issues (J. C. Rogers, 1983).

What is the Client's Current Status?

The first two things to determine are who is the client and what are the client's problem areas. Assessment of current status involves investigation beyond possible problem areas. The practitioner attempts to gain a total picture of the client: general health status, assets and limitations, strengths and weaknesses, needs, goals, values, beliefs, life style, and current life situation. It is only with such information that the client's problem areas can be truly understood. Assessment of motivation is also important, particularly when intervention is likely to be a lengthy process or when much of the problem resolution will require independent action on the part of the client.

Preassessment information regarding the client varies from none to considerable; considerable would include a health history, primary and secondary diagnoses, current physical and emotional status, and assessment summaries from other members of the health team. Starting with whatever information is available, the practitioner begins formulating a series of hypotheses about what the problem might be. Assessment focuses on collecting data that allow the hypotheses to be tested. The profession's applied body of knowledge serves as a guide for hypothesis formation, determining what data need to be collected and whether the data support or refute the hypotheses.

The process of hypothesis formation and testing continues until the practitioner is able to arrive at a reasonable conclusion, even if this conclusion may be based on insufficient data. The practitioner's conclusion may vary from finding no discernible problems, to identifying problem areas within the practitioner's domain of concern, to suspecting problems that are outside the practitioner's domain of concern.

As much as possible, the process of formulating

and testing hypotheses takes place in collaboration with the client. Nevertheless, practitioner and client may not always agree on the specific nature of the problem due to communication difficulties or to differences in values, perspective, and opinion. Discussion and negotiation are often helpful in reaching common agreement. When no agreement can be reached, the relationship usually ends.

What Can Be Done? With problems areas identified and with at least some understanding of the client as an individual, the practitioner considers available options for intervention. Sets of guidelines that address the problem areas provide information about options. Options usually are related to some kind of action, but the possibility of no intervention may also be entertained. Options are considered in the context of the individual client. With a list of options in hand, the practitioner compares them according to specific criteria: the probability of effectiveness (based on scientific evidence and/or clinical judgment); the time required to achieve the goals; the compatibility of the option with the client's situation; the impact of hazards, side effects, and economic considerations; and any other factors associated with an option that seem pertinent to the client. The practitioner essentially has a dialogue with himself or herself, considering and contrasting each of the options. On the basis of this process the practitioner discusses options with the client or client surrogate and makes recommendations. Discussion includes providing sufficient information to the client for informed decision making.

A word about clinical judgment: Judgment is the forming of an opinion, estimate, notion, or conclusion from available data. Used in conjunction with the word "clinical," judgment sometimes refers to arriving at a conclusion that goes beyond whatever scientific data are available. It involves the use of subjective impressions, one's general fund of knowledge, past experience, common sense, and, ideally, some wisdom.

What Will Be Done? A decision about problem resolution comes out of discussion between client and practitioner; the most feasible, acceptable option or options are selected. When appropriate, short- and long-term goals are set. As there may be several problem areas, a decision may need to be made about where to start. Occasionally, a practitioner and client cannot reach an agreement about any of the available options. The client may select other options that the practitioner cannot support. In such cases, the practitioner-client relationship is ended, at least for that time.

Although clinical reasoning and decision making have been described thus far as linear, the process is often circuitous. Problems may be identified incorrectly, additional problems may arise in the process of intervention, and the selected options may be found ineffective. The client may change his or her mind about a particular option in the course of intervention. For these and other reasons, clinical reasoning continues throughout intervention.

Because clinical reasoning and decision making are very human endeavors, there are possibilities for error. Practitioners may bring preconceived ideas about the client to reasoning/decision making, leading to misinterpreting data or ignoring data that do not support a favored hypothesis. Preferred options may be offered to a client without due consideration of other possibilities. Practitioners tend to remember only extreme cases, great successes, and spectacular failures, and forget the in-between times. Recommendations may also be made based on the assumption that the client is very much like the practitioner—an assumption that should never be entertained.

Practitioners tend to be problem oriented. More attention may be given to problem identification and selecting options for resolution than to the client as an individual. The client's general healthiness and abilities may be overlooked as well as his or her beliefs, values, and life style. Moreover, on the whole, practitioners tend to see more problems than are really present. Another facet of being problem-oriented is the tendency to see all problems as being within the client rather than in the client's environment. Two factors contribute to this tendency: (a) practitioners are likely to know more about the client than the environment and (b) the domains of concern and, thus, the applied bodies of knowledge of many professions are client-centered. Some professions have few, if any, sets of guidelines for practice dealing with problems located in the environment.

Finally, difficulties in problem resolution may be

related to how the client made the choices regarding the various options. The client may defer to the perceived wishes of the practitioner because the practitioner, as expert, is supposed to have the right answers. On the other hand, clients may not be able to make informed choices because of the nature of their problems or because of emotional states consequential to their problems. Thus, the practitioner must make sure the choices made by the client are indeed satisfactory to the client. Without mutual agreement, problem resolution may not proceed smoothly, if at all.

Although the process of clinical reasoning and decision making has been studied, much remains to be learned. It is unclear how it can be taught other than through apprenticeship experiences that foster imitation. No one seems to be certain whether it is primarily a logical process or an intuitive one. Finally, it is unknown how the clinical-reasoning and decision-making processes of one profession compare to another.

Some Problem Areas

Stated simply, the neopositivistic orientation views professions as having domains of concern and sets of guidelines for practice dealing with problems within their domain. In actuality, however, professions may have inadequate sets of guidelines—or none at all—for dealing with many problems. This situation is compounded by some practitioners' unwillingness to recognize this situation exists. Difficulties in practice may result.

Even after a reasonable amount of assessment and using various sets of guidelines for practice, practitioners are unable to identify a client's problems on occasion. When this is not recognized by the practitioner, he or she may unwittingly "bend" the available information in such a way so that it fits into a known category, a set of guidelines for practice. Real differences between the available information and the set of guidelines are ignored. When some small differences are recognized they may be dismissed as anomalies or as of no particular concern.

The above is an example of a practitioner not recognizing an *enigmatic problem*—a new or previously unobserved clinical problem for which there is no set of guidelines for practice (see Chapter 10 for further

Applied Scientific Inquiry in the Health Professions

elaboration). An example of a once-enigmatic problem is what we now refer to as AIDS, which was not initially recognized as a new disease or dealt with as such. Sometimes practitioners do recognize at some level that they are dealing with an enigmatic problem, but deal with the problem as if it were a known, understood problem. Sets of guidelines that are inappropriate to problem resolution are used.

Another difficulty is that ineffective sets of guidelines for practice may exist in a profession's applied body of knowledge. This is not the situation where there is general recognition that particular sets of guidelines are not very effective and continue to be used anyway because there is not sufficient theoretical knowledge to develop more effective sets of guidelines. Rather, the problem arises when the ineffectiveness of sets of guidelines goes unrecognized or ignored— for instance, using analytically oriented psychotherapy to assist individuals diagnosed with schizophrenia.

It should be noted that the difficulties just outlined are not the norm, although they probably occur in all of the health professions on occasion. Applied scientific inquiry is used continually to develop sets of guidelines for practice to deal with enigmatic problems. It is also used to update professions' applied bodies of knowledge through study, leading to refinement and further assessment of adequacy and to adding, retaining, and deleting sets of guidelines. Applied bodies of knowledge are always in a state of flux. Their overall adequacy is primarily dependent on the theoretical knowledge available. Adequacy, of course, is also dependent upon other resources—the time, money, and personnel the profession is able and willing to devote to applied scientific inquiry.

When practitioners recognize enigmatic problems in the immediacy of practice, they must deal with them as creatively as possible. Typically, practitioners engage in practical inquiry, drawing upon whatever imperfect knowledge is available and using trial and error to help resolve the problem. Attempts are often made to deal with peripheral problems for which there are adequate sets of guidelines for practice. While this is done with the full recognition that these attempts may well not resolve the central problem, the situation is approached with the hope that the central problem will be minimized. There are also times when practitioners decide that the best course of action is to do nothing.

When confronted with an enigmatic problem, attention must be turned to elucidating the problem, with the ultimate goal of developing an effective set of guidelines for practice. This process may require basic scientific inquiry and certainly requires applied scientific inquiry. Developing sets of guidelines for enigmatic problems is discussed in Section IV.

The Art of Practice

The art of practice is described separately from the perspectives of practice outlined above for two reasons. First, the art of practice is not directly related to sets of guidelines for practice. Second, a practitioner may be quite skilled in moving through the sequence of practice, using an applied body of knowledge, and in clinical reasoning and decision making, yet bring little or no art to practice.

In discussion of the phenomenological orientation, art of practice was described as skill in dealing with the uncertainty and individual-situation uniqueness found in practice (Schon, 1983). It was described as the essence of practice, the process involved in knowing and assisting a client. The art of practice is defined quite differently in the neopositivistic orientation (Blungart, 1973; Cassidy, 1962; Magraw, 1973).

Philosophers involved in the study of esthetics consider those qualities that allow objects and events to transcend the ordinary and become art. Typically, study of esthetics focuses on the literary, visual, and performing arts. This somewhat narrow perspective would seem to exclude daily human interactions from consideration. Such interactions, indeed, are often very ordinary and, at times, even offensive, but they also can be quite special. It is within the context of these latter interactions that one speaks of the art of practice in the neopositivistic orientation.

Practice that is art is any interaction that diminishes the isolation of the client, reaffirms the power of the human spirit, and assists the client in discovering meaning in existence. The art of practice contributes to fulfilling the universal need for kinship with others as well as for individuality. In experiencing the art of practice, clients identify with the human condition: the joys and sorrows, the sublime and ridiculous. Clients also feel their special ideas and concerns have been given recognition and substance.

The art of practice might be noticed only in retrospect. To use a fairly mundane example, a man leaves the dentist office after an unpleasant, painful experience with a lighter step, a small smile, and a feeling of being a bit more attractive. The man feels better, not physically, but inside himself. He has experienced the art of practice.

The art of practice is shared by all health professions and, as far as we know, is the same for all health professions. The art of practice is not related to a profession's applied body of knowledge, however it is defined, or to a profession's philosophical assumptions. The beliefs, values, and goals of all health professions support, indeed encourage, the art of practice. One of the major problems in discussing the art of practice is its elusive nature. Little is known about the art of practice—what exactly it is and how it is learned—though few would deny its existence and importance. Nevertheless, some aspects of the art of practice can be described.

One component of the art of practice is the practitioner's ability to perceive the uniqueness or specialness of each individual. Paradoxically, the practitioner must also be able to perceive universality—the individual as a member of the human community and participant in the human condition. The differentness of each individual and the similarities of all individuals are recognized at once. Another component of the art of practice is perception of the individual as indivisible, as an integrated whole, not a collection of parts or systems. Although intervention may focus on one particular problem area, a specific person has the problem. The person is not attached to a problem; rather, the problem is integral to the person. Individuals cannot be divided. A third component of the art of practice is recognition of the rights and dignity of each person. Much has been written about the rights of clients to be adequately informed, to make choices, to reject treatment, and so on. Less has been written about dignity. Recognition of dignity involves being respectful of the individual's person as well as his or her beliefs and values. It involves acting in a decorous manner with the degree of formality and gravity the situation requires. Through the recognition of dignity, honor is given to each client.

Formality and gravity are part of the art of practice, but so too is joy and humor. A practitioner's recognition of the ridiculous in the human condition gives perspective to the serious and painful. The capacity to sometimes "be at play" may provide respite from the mundane and boring. Humor has universal elements, joining an individual with many others. But it may also be something very private between client and practitioner—a shared joke, a memory of a ludicrous incident—that marks the uniqueness of the client's experience.

The capacity to empathize is another component of the art of practice. Empathy involves entering into the experience of another person without losing one's own sense of separateness as an individual. It is the ability to feel the pain and joy of another person, yet fully realizing it is not one's own pain and joy. Empathy enables one to understand on an emotional rather than only an intellectual level, but the separateness of empathy is also important as it enables the practitioner to be objective and make sound judgments. The togetherness and separateness of empathy are of equal importance, two sides of one coin.

The components outlined above give only a partial view of the art of practice. Other components could be added; the list is probably quite lengthy. But even with a very long list, a definitive definition is unlikely to emerge. We often know when we have been the recipient of the art of practice; we are sometimes aware of engaging in the art of practice. But despite all of that knowledge, the art of practice remains a mysterious process. Because of the recondite nature of the art of practice, it cannot be directly taught although it is probably a learned process. We may experience its development in ourselves and observe its growth in students and colleagues. Although the art of practice cannot be directly taught, once perceived in ourselves or others we can nurture its growth.

In the neopositivistic orientation, the art of practice is seen as very distinct from the skilled use of knowledge. The knowledgeable and skilled practitioner is able to select appropriate sets of guidelines for practice to assist each client with his or her problems, and he or she knows when there are no appropriate sets of guidelines. The knowledgeable and skilled practitioner is able to interpret conflicting data, make sound decisions based on less then adequate information, and take those intuitive leaps that lead to new understanding. None of this is the art of practice, however.

At times in the literature, the term, "art of practice," refers to acting without sufficient knowledge or to improvising and creatively using trial and error. "Art of practice" is also used as a euphemism for lack of knowledge. Science and art are viewed as being on a continuum ranging from practice based on theoretically sound, effective sets of guidelines (science) to working pretty much in the dark (art). But this, too, is not the art of practice as described here.

Neopositivists recognize the need to work outside of sets of guidelines for practice and the inadequacy of some sets of guidelines that are used. Through such recognition, applied scientific inquiry is prompted and fostered. Lack of knowledge is never confused with the art of practice, nor is the art of practice seen as a substitute for knowledge.

Whereas science may be used to mend the body and mind, it is the art of practice that mends the spirit.

Section III:
Basic Scientific Inquiry

The previous section provided an overview of the neopositivistic epistemological orientation to practice. Since practice in this orientation is founded on theory and empirical data, this section focuses on theoretical information and the process whereby theoretical information is developed—basic scientific inquiry. Theory is emphasized because it is the ultimate and desired end product of basic scientific inquiry.

6. *Theory and Basic Scientific Inquiry*

The first section of this chapter, primarily introductory in nature, is concerned with two issues: (a) why there is a need to understand theory and what about it needs to be understood, and (b) why there is general discomfort with theory in the health professions. Various possible reasons for this discomfort are identified.

The evolution of basic science and its separation from philosophy began in the 16th century. Over the next several hundred years, science evolved into a particular type of scholarly inquiry with its own unique characteristics. Scientific inquiry is also a very human endeavor subject to the dynamics of people working together and the influence of the society in which it takes place. These two aspects of science are addressed in the second and third sections of this chapter.

Understanding Theory
The Need To Understand

In order to engage in applied scientific inquiry—to formulate, refine, and assess the adequacy of sets of guidelines for practice—applied scientists must have a firm grasp of theory. They must know what it is and how it is developed, tested, and refined.

In a sense, applied scientists have more to learn than basic scientists. The latter have only to master the process of basic scientific inquiry. They have little, if any, need to understand applied scientific inquiry because it is not within their domain. While some basic scientists—particularly those who work closely with applied scientists—are concerned about applied scientific inquiry, they do not need to master the process of applied scientific inquiry. Applied scientists, on the other hand, must be knowledgeable about both basic and applied inquiry.

An understanding of theory provides the foundation for two of the major concerns of applied scientists. The first concern is the question of whether a particular theory is suitable for use as the basis, in whole or in part, for a set of guidelines for practice. In order to answer that question, the applied scientist must know what constitutes the content and structure of theory and how the validity of theory is determined. In addition, the applied scientist must be able to compare different theories concerned with the same phenomena in order to decide which is more suitable for a particular set of guidelines.

The second concern of applied scientists is the need to extrapolate from theory. Extrapolation involves many processes, some of which require taking elements out of theories, reformulating these elements, and combining them with elements from other theories. Theories do not break when dismantled; nevertheless, they must be taken apart with care in order to preserve the meaning and essence of the detached elements. This can only be done successfully when one has full understanding of the nature of theory.

Although understanding theory is necessary for those concerned with developing sets of guidelines for practice, it is also important for those involved in their use. Sets of guidelines for practice can be employed effectively without an understanding of theory, but the practitioner is then functioning on a technical rather than a professional level. Knowledge of the nature of theory and of how sets of guidelines are formulated through the use of theory help the practitioner to understand the purpose of sets of guidelines, the advantage of their use as the basis for practice, and their limitations. Using sets of guidelines for practice without understanding theory is like driving a car without knowing anything about its internal mechanism and proper maintenance. It is fine when the car works, but when it does not, one is left in a total quandary, unable to proceed to the desired destination.

There is one additional reason for understanding theory and how theory is developed, tested, and refined. In working with clients, the practitioner may be confronted with phenomena that have not been subjected to basic scientific inquiry and about which there are no theories or empirical data. When this happens, the practitioner must turn to an appropriate scientific discipline to request the development of theory. This is exemplified by medicine turning to the various biological sciences for knowledge about the causal factors of AIDS.

In order to request development of theoretical knowledge, practitioners must have a reasonable understanding of what theory is. Without this understanding, they would be unable to clearly state what exactly they need. Because practitioners may be literally at a loss for words when attempting the language of basic scientific inquiry, working with basic scientists may seem frightening and, thus, be avoided. Such reactions are a serious detriment to a profession's continued viability.

Discomfort with Theory

For many in the health professions, one of the factors that impedes understanding of basic scientific inquiry—and, by extension, applied inquiry—is a general sense of discomfort with theory. The biggest problem is the way theory is taught in professional education. "Theory" is usually not defined. Attention is given to the content of theory only; the origin, structure, and function of theory are rarely discussed. Human anatomy, for example, is considered in great detail, but few students realize they are studying a theory. Theories labeled as such—for instance, "theories leadership"—are recognized as theories only due to their titles, not to understanding. The differences and relationship between theory and empirical data are infrequently addressed.

With some exceptions, theories are usually not taught in their complete and original form. Rather, truncated versions or summaries are provided for consideration. In the study of human development, for example, students study a synthesis of several theories with little if any awareness of the theories that have been combined.

Theories studied in the course of a professional education are usually only those considered to be basic to the profession's practice, which seems reasonable given the purpose and time constraints of professional education. However, the drawback to such an approach is that students rarely have an opportunity to explore why some theories are fundamental to the profession's practice and others are not. The question simply is not raised.

Students seldom have an opportunity to play with theories. Content is to be learned or memorized. The spirit of play is not encouraged. Theories are not taken apart, compared with other theories, examined from a variety of perspectives, combined with other theories, or considered relative to one's self. Without a playful approach to theories, students are ill-prepared to engage in applied scientific inquiry. It is like expecting a child to be able to construct an elaborate house of blocks when the child has never played with them before.

The term "theory" is often used loosely in professional education, referring to such nontheory concepts as empirical data, sets of guidelines for practice, taxonomies, single postulates, philosophical statements, and so forth. At times, the term is used in the lay sense of a conjecture or speculation about some phenomena. This vagueness of definition can be confusing to students.

Finally, the way basic scientific inquiry is taught in professional education is often detrimental to understanding theory. Course work is typically directed toward mastery of research designs—agreed-upon, formalized strategies of science used for gathering quantitative and qualitative data and for treating that data. Little attention is given to the study of basic scientific inquiry itself (Kerlinger, 1960; Williams, 1974a). Moreover, the relationship between research design and developing, testing, and refining theory is often not emphasized. The problem may be compounded by no clear distinction being made between basic and applied scientific inquiry.

For at least some of the reasons outlined above, many practitioners are uncomfortable with theory. They are not sure what it is, where it comes from, or even how one goes about reading theory. Lack of such knowledge may lead to a sense that it is too complicated for comprehension. Such a situation is not conducive to the understanding of basic scientific inquiry or the ultimate mastery of applied scientific inquiry.

The remainder of this chapter and the next two chapters provide an orientation to theory and the process of basic scientific inquiry. Admittedly, one purpose is to limit or interrupt any possible phobic response to theory. More positively, however, the purpose is to help the reader to gain sufficient understanding of theory so that it becomes a known entity, familiar, and comfortable to be with.

Characteristics of Basic Science

Basic science has several characteristics that distinguish it from the other forms of inquiry—such as philosophical inquiry, historical inquiry, and practical inquiry. Seven of these characteristics are described here (Gould, 1989; Kerlinger, 1986; Lowe, 1962; Popper, 1968; Shapere, 1984; Singleton, Straits, Straits, & McAllister, 1988).

The fundamental assumptions of science.

Scientists believe that the physical universe has order and that such order can be known without recourse to supernatural explanation. They believe logical reasoning, observation, and verification of observation will lead to understanding the physical universe.

The singular goal of basic scientific inquiry is to gain greater knowledge.

Basic science is about seeking knowledge—to make what is unknown, known. The search is paramount, leading wherever it goes, with no strictures on what can be known or should be known. Basic science is driven by curiosity and, for some, by the need to find general principles that describe the physical universe.

On occasion, basic scientific inquiry may be directed toward practical ends—that is, particular theoretical information may be sought in order to solve a given practical problem. In this situation, basic scientists are guided by applied scientists. The latter usually determines what needs to be known and whether particular lines of inquiry are likely to lead to information that can be used. Basic scientists follow only those lines of inquiry that seem fruitful for the immediate purpose. Other lines of inquiry that may lead to new knowledge are set aside—to be investigated at another time.

Basic science guided by applied science usually occurs in a situation of perceived urgency. A classic example is the basic scientific inquiry that took place to provide a theoretical foundation for developing the vaccine for poliomyelitis. The goal and processes of basic science do not change in such a situation. Moreover, applied science leading basic science is acceptable only under temporary circumstances; in the long run, it is seen as detrimental to the development of new theoretical knowledge. Basic scientific inquiry is usually most productive when it is allowed to move in whatever direction investigation leads, unimpeded by the need for specific information required to serve as the foundation for solving a practical problem.

Basic science organizes knowledge into the structure of theory.

Basic scientists seek order and are most comfortable when knowledge is ordered in the form of a theory. Nevertheless, some theoretical knowledge may initially be in the form of empirical data or postulates that identify the relationship between two or more concepts. These postulates are "free floating" in that they have not yet been incorporated into the formal structure of a theory. Other theoretical knowledge may be in the form of taxonomies—conceptual systems that order phenomena into different categories and according to various levels of abstraction. Development of a taxonomy is sometimes the first step in theory development.

Basic science relies on preplanned and controlled study.

Although scientists play with ideas and tinker with objects, this play ultimately leads to study based on a predetermined scheme that provides for necessary controls. The plan may be revised repeatedly, but there is always a plan. Although new knowledge is sometimes gained through fortuitous happenings, before such knowledge is presented to the scientific community it must be subjected to preplanned and controlled study in order to be credible.

Basic science is grounded in documented evidence.

Research designs and findings used to arrive at theoretical statements are the evidence of science. Documentation takes place during the process of inquiry and is reported afterwards. The present stylized way of writing research reports has evolved out of the need to present sufficient documented evidence to support theoretical statements. This documentation allows for the verification of observation—a hallmark of basic science. The demand for documented evidence was one of the factors contributing to the separation of science from the theologically centered philosophy of the 16th century. Science was to be based on data available for all to see, not on authority or faith.

Science is fallible and liable to error, falseness, and inaccuracy.

Scientific findings and theories are always considered provisional. Regardless of how often and elegantly a particular theory has been tested and found to have a high degree of validity, it is always considered tentative. All theoretical information remains open to continued assessment by contemporary and future scientists. The edict "to question what is known" is taken seriously by scientists; they do not speak of "proof" or "truth." Although theories can be demonstrated to be invalid, they can never be proven. Moreover, it is not the business of science to seek truth; that task is for philosophers and theologians.

It is difficult for some people to accept the fallibility of science. Although there is recognition that past theories have been inaccurate—for instance, illness is caused by the imbalance of the four humors or schizophrenia is an intrapsychic problem—there tends to be a belief that the current theories are accurate. Many seem to think, "now we are smarter; now we know." People thought the same way 40 years ago—and 400 years ago.

Science has an evolving code of ethics.

Traditionally, two ethical principles have guided scientific inquiry: (a) to represent one's own work accurately and honestly and (b) to give adequate credit to the work of others. Over the past 30 years, the code of ethics governing scientific inquiry has been expanded to cover many more specific aspects of inquiry—primarily with the intent to protect human participants, animal subjects, and the physical environment. Abuse in these areas was so widespread that additional principles and rules of conduct needed to be developed and formalized. Most proposed scientific inquiry must now be approved by some type of review board to ensure adherence to ethical principles. The scientific community is also much more aware of the need for continuing study and articulation of ethical principles to guide inquiry into new areas.

Science has a strong tradition of communication.

Almost from the inception of basic science, societies were formed and journals developed for the purpose of sharing information. Scientists continue to be aware of the importance of communication in the search for theoretical knowledge because they realize that they are most productive when they are able to draw on the resources of past and current scientific activity. Indeed, the history of science is the story of how scientists have built upon the work of others distant from them in time and place. The tradition of sharing the process and product of individual projects of inquiry is deeply ingrained in science.

These outlined characteristics of basic scientific inquiry are accepted by the vast majority of scientists. The characteristics are ideals, but ideals that scientists see as very much a part of their work. Nevertheless, because science is a very human endeavor, the ideal is not always the real.

A Human Endeavor

Until the recent past, basic scientific inquiry has been universally viewed as an exemplary occupation engaged in by dedicated individuals who were above reproach. Basic scientists were set apart, placed on a higher level somehow above those in other occupations. Members of the various scientific disciplines were also viewed as being isolated from society, unaffected by its beliefs and not required to be held accountable by it.

It is now recognized that basic scientific inquiry is very much a part of the society in which it takes place (Degler, 1991; Diesing, 1982; Grove, 1989; Kneller, 1978; Kuhn, 1970; Perutz, 1989; Regis, 1987; Rosenberg, 1976; Shapere, 1984). The beliefs and values of a society influence the extent to which basic scientific inquiry is seen as an acceptable and valued activity. Society also determines the extent to which scientists are free to pursue desired lines of inquiry and the share of a society's economic resources allotted to basic inquiry.

At the present time, societies typically control basic science—including the phenomena studied and the research designs—through the allocation of public funds and, to a lesser extent, private funds. Scientists can only afford to study phenomena and use research designs for which funds are available. The extent to which the current, fairly extensive control of basic science by society helps or hinders the search for knowledge is not known.

The values and beliefs of society also influence science in other, more subtle ways. This is exemplified quite nicely by considering how Charles Darwin's theory of biological evolution has been interpreted (Degler, 1991). Although his theory was developed by at least 1842, Darwin did not publish *On the Origin of the Species* until 1859 primarily because of his well-founded belief that the theory would cause public outcry and consternation in the scientific community. Later, Darwin's theory influenced the interpretation of sociological and psychological data to support a common belief of the day—the superiority of white, Anglo- Saxon men and the society they had created. Sometimes referred to as social Darwinism or social evolution, this theory was used as a rationale for all sorts of social activities now recognized as inhumane, the repression of women and colonialism to name two. This was done without any serious objection from social scientists because social Darwinism was considered to be a valid theory.

Social Darwinism, now recognized as invalid, is an extreme example. However, the values and beliefs of society have influenced—and always will influence—basic science. Basic science is not a value-free activity. Contemporary illustrations of the influence of values on basic science can be seen in studies that touch on issues of the equality of the sexes. For example, several studies have indicated that strenuous physical exercise is detrimental to the reproduction processes and the maintenance of adequate bone calcium in young women. Until recently, these studies were dismissed as being simply sexually biased interpretations of data. Another example is the difficulty that both scientists and lay people have in entertaining the idea that differences in quantitative reasoning between men and women may be biologically based rather than due to social factors.

Society influences scientific communication. Although the tradition of science dictates open communication, society may see such communication as detrimental to its well-being—especially concerning information that has potential for enhancing a society's military or economic power. It should also be noted that communication may be limited by individuals or small groups of scientists for a period of time in order to enhance their own honor, glory, and perhaps financial gain. Again, it is not known whether the advancement of knowledge is hindered by societal or individual limits placed on communication.

A concerned society influences the ethical principles operant in scientific inquiry. Many lay people play a major role in developing ethical standards to protect people, animals, and the environment. Society as represented by the government periodically becomes concerned about the degree of honesty and integrity in the scientific community (Gould, 1989; Hilts, 1991). Sloppiness and false reporting of research designs and findings have been found in the work of some scientists. Whether this represents a problem with a select few or with many is unknown. Nevertheless, the government continues to seek ways to minimize such blatant disregard for ethical standards regarding accuracy and honesty in reporting scientific information.

Some sectors of the scientific community have been concerned about developing and enforcing their own ethical standards. And while a few scientists have taken the leadership in this area, the general culture of the scientific community tends to impede self-examination and regulation. The culture of science is characterized, in part, by a laissez-faire attitude—noninterference in the affairs of others, particularly with reference to individual conduct and or freedom of action (Flexner & Hauck, 1987). There is a belief within the scientific community that all scientists behave in an ethical manner. To question another scientist's ethics is considered both unnecessary and unacceptable. In general, research design and findings are accepted as presented. Although studies are repeated by others, this is done primarily for the purpose of verification, not to determine whether a report is false. The work of others may be questioned privately among a small group of colleagues, but rarely in a public forum. This laissez-faire attitude is one of the reasons society has had to take such an active role in questioning the activities of scientists.

Basic scientists also misrepresent the goal of basic scientific inquiry. Basic science is *not* concerned with control of the physical universe or the betterment of the lot of humankind. These two goals are in the domain of applied science. However, almost since science distinguished itself from philosophy, basic scientists have sought financial support for their work—from patrons, government, and industry—using eloquent statements about the potential practical application of whatever inquiry is being proposed. In so doing, supplicants are often being dishonest. No one can know what knowledge will be discovered or if such knowledge will have any use. Moreover, basic scientists rarely have the ability to translate theoretical information into useful sets of guidelines for action, nor are they interested in doing so. This tradition of misrepresentation of the goal of basic scientific inquiry is troubling because it leaves the public with a false understanding of basic scientific inquiry. This is nowhere more evident than in the time required for beginning students to shed their inaccurate ideas about the goals of basic scientific inquiry and, by extension, of applied inquiry.

Despite this predominant laissez-faire attitude, the culture of science is also characterized by authoritarianism—power in the hands of a few. A few members of a scientific discipline control the financial resources available to the discipline as a whole, as well as the access to public forums: journals, conference presentations, major meetings, and symposia. Perhaps more significantly, the select few of each discipline tend to dictate what phenomena will be studied and what theories tested. Phenomena and theories not considered relevant by those in authority may be ignored. Findings that do not support the favored theory or theories likewise may be given little attention or even severely criticized. Indeed, a favored theory may be studied long after it is apparent to outside observers that the theory is woefully inadequate. The Big Bang theory of the universe's creation, for example, is a highly favored theory but one that, as currently stated, does not account for a number of observed phenomena (Burbidge, 1992).

When a discipline does accept the inadequacy of a predominant or major theory, a search begins for a potentially more adequate theory. Kuhn (1970) refers to this as a crisis period, a turning point in a discipline. A crisis period is characterized by considerable conflict and shifting alliances. The new theory that gains favor may not be the one that has the most potential for describing, and allowing for, accurate prediction about the phenomena in question. According to Kuhn, it seems to be more a matter of who is the most successful in the struggle for power.

The authoritarianism of basic science is somewhat surprising. One of the factors prompting the development of modern science was the move away from the authoritarianism of the Church. The physical universe was to be studied through observation and logical reasoning, not influenced by the beliefs of those in authority. On the other hand, some people are more comfortable working within an authoritarian structure, and the desire for power is very human.

Lest the reader who is a member of a health profession begin to feel smug, most professions also have a culture characterized by a mixture of laissez-faire and authoritarianism. The problems inherent in working in a broader culture also plague professions.

7. *The Methods of Science*

T he methods of science are those intellectual activities involved in doing scientific inquiry. They are not unique to science but, rather, are methods used in many types of scholarly inquiry, including esthetic or historical, for example. The methods of science are described in relation to the phenomena to which they are addressed—the physical universe.

The methods of science should not be confused with research designs, which are the agreed-upon, formalized strategies used for gathering and treating quantitative and qualitative data. The methods of science are used irrespective of research design and within and outside of the context of employing research designs. The intellectual activities of science take place throughout the process of inquiry, whereas research, as the term is usually used, is limited to part of the process. Research designs are not discussed here because there are many other excellent texts on the subject. These texts tend to give far less attention to the methods of science, however.

The methods of science are used in both basic and applied inquiry. The description here focuses more on the methods of basic inquiry in order to assist the reader in understanding basic scientific inquiry, an understanding that is fundamental to applied inquiry.[1]

---

[1] The methods of science described draw upon the work of Broudy, Ennis, and Krimerman (1973), Goldstein (1988), Grove (1989), Kerlinger (1986), Marx and Cronan-Hillix (1987), Popper (1968), Singleton, Straits, Straits, and McAllister (1988), and Vockell (1983).

Although each method of science is considered individually, there is frequent overlap between them. For example, categorizing and defining are in some ways two aspects of the same process. Moreover, some intellectual activities—like speculation and judgment—take place simultaneously so that it is difficult to separate one from the other. The methods of science have been placed in four categories, roughly following the sequence of investigation.

The Fundamentals

One of the assumptions of rational empiricism is that the physical universe can become known through the combined use of the processes of observation and logical reasoning. The other methods to be described here are in many ways either components of observation or logical reasoning or involve a combination of the two. Thus, observation and logical reasoning are fundamental to an understanding of the methods of science.

Observation

Observation is the process of regarding with attention for the purpose of noting the characteristics of phenomena. Observation may be systematized in that the observer is looking for or at particular characteristics in an organized manner—often assisted by various research designs. On the other hand, if the observation is unsystematized, the observer is not looking for any particular characteristic. Rather, he or she attempts to be as unselective as possible and notes all the characteristics of the phenomena, as well as what characteristics are absent.

Observation in science tends to move from being unsystematized toward being systematized. Regardless of how systematized observation may be, there is always an attempt "to observe what is not being observed." Often, in the process of highly systematized observation, important but seemingly irrelevant characteristics of the phenomena are first noted. Good scientists are always observant even when they are far from the business of science. Observation becomes an ingrained, lifelong habit.

Observation is often thought of as attending to phenomena—people, events, and things—external to the self. However, observation also includes attending to one's own feelings, ideas, and experiences. Self-

Applied Scientific Inquiry in the Health Professions

observation has been the initial source of many theories in the social sciences, particularly psychology. Perhaps the best known example is Freud's use of his dreams and fantasies in the development of psychoanalytic theory.

Observation is also the process basic to *review of the literature*. Consideration of what others have observed—their speculations, research designs, and interpretations of findings—is an important part of scientific inquiry. Scientists should be able to contemplate their ideas and particular observations in the context of a broader body of knowledge. Science advances through the expansion of the literature—an individual's work building on the work of others. Although reviewing the literature is essential to scientific inquiry, it may sometimes impede it. First, people tend to believe that the interpretations of research findings that they read are the only possible interpretations. When one's observations are incompatible with the published views of others, one may question oneself rather than the literature. Second, the literature often presents phenomena from a limited number of perspectives. The perspective of the literature frequently becomes the filter through which the reader makes his or her subsequent observations. The bias so formed may influence what is observed. To be both conversant with the literature while at the same time being a naive observer is often a difficult feat to accomplish.

Logical Reasoning

Logical reasoning is the process of forming a conclusion based on premises with information used as evidence. It requires strict attention to evidence and to how conclusions are derived from evidence. Two forms of logical reasoning are usually described—deductive and inductive.

In deductive reasoning the conclusion follows necessarily from the premises on which it is based—that is, if one uses only the premises provided, no other conclusion can be drawn. The following syllogism is an example of deductive reasoning:

1. All horses are animals (premise).

2. Lester is a horse (premise).

3. Therefore, Lester is an animal (conclusion).

In deductive reasoning one is first concerned with whether the premises and the conclusion are "true" or "false." That is, given the limits of all knowledge, are they accurate or inaccurate, plausible or implausible? Second, one is concerned with the validity of the argument. A valid argument is one in which the conclusion is based on, and only on, the evidence provided. When the premises and the conclusion are judged to be true and the argument valid, a process of deductive reasoning is said to be sound. Sound deductive reasoning ultimately provides support for the knowledge generated by science.

The other form of logical reasoning is inductive. In this reasoning process, conclusions are proposed that go beyond the evidence presented in the premises. Thus, no matter how accurate or plausible the evidence, the conclusion is always considered tentative. An example of inductive reasoning is:

1. I hear the sound of thunder and automobile tires swishing on wet pavement.
2. It was cloudy when I came inside.
3. Therefore, it is raining.

The conclusion here may be true. However, it might not be raining; the street could have just been washed. In considering a conclusion drawn from inductive reasoning, other plausible conclusions are always entertained.

Inductive reasoning is one of the major forces affecting science, leading to the formulation of new hypotheses and taking science beyond what is known. For many, the fun of science is in inductive reasoning and following where the reasoning leads. It should be noted, however, that both deductive and inductive reasoning are important parts of scientific inquiry and necessary for its success.

Toward the Task at Hand

The "task" of concern here may be the doing of basic or applied scientific inquiry. There is some sense of sequence implied in the following methods of science. But in reality, inquiry is often far more circuitous than linear.

Formulating Questions

A question is an interrogatory statement formulated for the purpose of gaining information about any matter involving uncertainty or doubt. Questions give essential direction to the process of scientific inquiry. A given scientific question influences all that follows—the data to be gathered, what is done with the data, and interpretation of the findings. Questions are a statement of the work to be done. A good scientific question is precisely stated, clearly focused, and without need of a preamble in order to be comprehended. When such a question is posed, a major part of any project has been completed; the task ahead is clearly demarcated, and one is halfway home, so to speak. Formulating a good question is often a lengthy process, frequently preceded by developing, refining, and discarding many tentative questions. By so doing, a definitive question is created that can be used to guide more in-depth inquiry. Formulating questions is more than just an attempt to develop a "good" question, however; it is a way of thinking that permeates all of scientific inquiry. Scientists raise questions, entertain questions, and talk about questions. What, where, when, and how are the dominant words in the vocabulary of science. While scientists are working on one question, other questions are usually raised. A scientist without questions is a very unhappy scientist (Feynman, 1985).

Collecting Data

Data collection is the process of gathering pieces of information for the purpose of answering a question. What data and how the data are gathered depends largely on the question posed. The process of gathering data may be highly systemized, rigorously delimited by a given type of research design. On the other hand, data collection may be relatively unsystematized, guided more by opportunity and what becomes available in the process of data collection. How systematic the data collection is depends on many factors, including the questions posed, the type of research design being used, the nature of the phenomena, and the tools available for gathering data.

As in the case of the formulation of questions, data collection is an habitual activity for scientists. There is the formal assembling of data, systematized or unsystematized, but there are also the odd pieces of information that are gathered. The file cabinets of many scientists are full of data noticed in casual observation, inadvertently generated by chance, or saved as an artifact of a research project. Such data may not be used immediately because of the constraints of time or because an adequate question has not been posed. The data are happily squirrelled away for future use.

Analyzing

Analysis is the process of separating a phenomenon into constituent parts or elements, usually for some predetermined purpose. The purpose of an analysis is all important because it determines how the parts of the whole will be divided and considered.

The process of an analysis is based ultimately on a system or framework of analytical concepts—concepts used to identify elements of a whole. Some simple examples of analytical concepts are hue, shade, and tone or structure, function, and content. The framework selected is strongly influenced by the purpose of analysis. For example, one may analyze a painting to identify either the school to which it belongs or the type of media used to create it. Although there might be some overlap in analysis, the conceptual framework used to determine the painting's origin would be different than the one employed for an analysis of the type of media used.

It is quite difficult to analyze an entity without some kind of conceptual framework. If one were asked to analyze a chair, without any other directions, there would likely be a long pause. How should the task be approached? Should one consider the parts, the materials used in construction, its possible functions, or its esthetic appeal?

A framework for analysis may be chosen prior to analysis. For example, the periodic table of elements is usually used to analyze the components of an unknown substance. On the other hand, an analytic framework may be developed subsequent to a preliminary study of the phenomena because the purpose may not be clear. To illustrate, prior to formal study of low birth weight three-year-old children, a group of scientists observes such children to determine what factors to consider. Only after such an observation do they decide that cognitive function will be the subject of the study. With their purpose now clear, they either select an existing conceptual framework for analysis of cognitive function, or they develop one specifically suited to their investigation.

Analysis should not be confused with reductionism—the belief that complex phenomena are best understood through study of the simplest, most basic mechanisms operant in the phenomena. Analysis is a process; reductionism is a belief about the proper focus of scientific inquiry. Analysis occurs in science regardless of whether larger or smaller units are considered appropriate for study.

In some of the health professions, "reductionism" has been transformed into meaning only devoting attention to clients' problems and not being concerned about clients as individuals. This is a misrepresentation of reductionism and is detrimental to the understanding both of scientific inquiry and of how we can become more sensitive to the individual needs of clients.

Synthesizing   Synthesis, the opposite of analysis, is the process of combining elements into a single, unified whole. The purpose of synthesis is important because—like analysis—it determines what elements will be used in a process and how they will be combined. Synthesis may occur by happenstance or through trial and error, but, more typically, some goal, idea, or conceptual system is used as a guide. Examples of synthesis include making a skirt, preparing a meal, and some aspects of developing sets of guidelines for practice.

The analysis and synthesis that occur in habitual activities are often so intimately connected that one tends to fade into the other. In evaluation with a client, for example, behavior is observed, essential elements of that behavior are noted (analysis), and from that information a client's problems areas are identified (synthesis). The practitioner may have difficulty sorting out just what was analysis and what was synthesis.

Synthesis is rarely discussed in the scientific literature. The term "analysis" is used far more often, and it frequently seems to denote both analysis and synthesis. Consider the term "data analysis." Data are indeed analyzed in this process, but determining the mean and standard deviation, for example, is to a great extent a process of synthesis, not analysis. In qualitative research, we speak of "analyzing the data to identify common themes," but certainly a good deal of synthesis must take place also.

The point is that synthesis is an essential part of scientific inquiry. In labeling the process improperly, we tend to ignore synthesis relative to both studying the process and learning how to engage in it. Analysis without synthesis is a meaningless process, comparable to stating premises without drawing any conclusions. The task has not been completed. Conversely, synthesis without analysis could be compared to arriving at a conclusion without any premises.

Categorizing   Categorizing is the process of arranging phenomena into groups or of classifying phenomena in some manner. Basic science is founded on the study of particular individual phenomena. Theories, however, are about categories of phenomena, not a single phenomenon. Thus, commonalities across and among phenomena must be identified prior to theory development. Individual entities with like characteristics are grouped together to form a category. These categories—or, to use the language of science, concepts—are one of the three structural elements of theory.

Categories are so much a part of language and our way of perceiving the world that they are sometimes difficult to understand. You, the individual reader, are a single entity, but I have placed you in a category, "reader," with all the other individual readers. You could also be placed in other categories: woman, practitioner, student, Chinese, hungry, bored, or liberal. Any single entity can usually be placed in a variety of categories. The thing that contains my coffee is not just a cup; it is a container, ceramic, breakable, and so forth.

For lay people, the process of categorizing is often unconscious. We are born into a culture with categories that become our own. And new categories are frequently added, for instance, software, word processing, creationism, right-to-life, and the ever-changing language of adolescents. The meaning of new categories is learned by us as individuals, yet we have not really engaged in the process of categorizing.

To get a feeling for the process of categorizing, imagine the first anatomists who engaged in human

Applied Scientific Inquiry in the Health Professions

dissection. There was much to categorize. Common characteristics as well as distinct differences needed to be identified before categories such as arteries and veins, ligaments and tendons, and bone and cartilage could be created.

Categories may be generally shared by members of a large cultural group or only by a minority—a particular community, an age group, or even one high school. The jargon of a particular discipline or profession may be almost incomprehensible because the categories used are unknown to the outsider. Finally, categories may be shared by a few people such as a circle of friends or members of a family. In the author's family of origin, for example, household tasks were categorized as "boy jobs" and "girl jobs." Sexist as it may seem now, this categorization excused the author from a number of onerous tasks.

Defining

A category remains a private matter and useless to others until it is defined. Defining is the process of describing the essential characteristics and fixing the boundaries of a given category. Defining is often more difficult than it seems at first glance, especially when distinguishing between characteristics that are essential and those that are merely present but are not vital. Think for a moment of defining "chair." What are the essential characteristics necessary to describe "chairness," and to differentiate "chair" from "stool" or "bench?"

Much of scientific inquiry involves formulating and reformulating definitions. Without adequate definitions, inquiry can proceed only so far, impeded by lack of agreement on what constitutes a particular category. For example, because there is no common agreement on the definition of "spasticity," what two scientists consider spasticity may not be the same. Such vagueness impedes research and the pooling of research findings. The latter is particularly important because greater understanding is gained and theories are developed only through the combination of research findings from a variety of projects.

Defining and categorizing are interrelated processes. In the process of categorizing, tentative definitions are formulated. As a category becomes more refined and fixed, so too does the definition. While the processes are often so intermingled that it may be difficult for the observer or formulator to distinguish one from the other, the processes are different and of equal importance. Definitions are also one of the structural elements of theory. They and the process of defining are discussed in greater detail in the description of theory.

Seeking Relationships

Seeking relationships is the process of determining whether two or more categories of phenomena are associated and what the nature of that association might be. Basic science is concerned first with describing, categorizing, and defining, but it seeks to go beyond that level of knowledge to the level of determining and predicting the relationships between phenomena.

Relationships between phenomena are sought through observation, analysis, and logical reasoning. Relationships are identified through synthesis. Identifying relationships may be augmented by the use of various types of quantitative research designs involving the manipulation of phenomena and measurement and the use of statistics. However, qualitative research designs, which do not involve such activities, are also used in the process of seeking relationships.

The terms "descriptive" and "predictive" are used in science to refer both to the status of a field of study and to theories. Descriptive refers to knowledge of the characteristics of isolated categories of phenomena. Predictive refers to understanding how phenomena interact to such an extent that knowledge of one phenomenon enables one to predict how another phenomenon will react or behave. The line between descriptive and predictive theories is not firm; the difference is often a matter of degree rather than kind. For example, human anatomy is usually thought of as a descriptive theory for it describes the structures of the human body, yet human anatomy is also a predictive theory as every surgeon demonstrates.

Prediction should not be confused with determining the "why" of a relationship. Science is not concerned with answering "why?" That question is not in its domain. We know, for example, that matter behaves in various ways, and we can make fairly accurate predictions about the behavior of some matter in certain circumstances. But, ultimately, we really do not know why matter behaves in that manner. Similarly, we do not know why positive reinforcement is effective in altering some kinds of behavior or why the HIV virus attacks the immune system. Basic scientists are only concerned with gaining sufficient knowledge to accurately predict that A and only A, under circumstances X and Y, will lead to B and only B.

In science, the relationships between categories of phenomena are referred to as postulates, the third structural element of theory. They too will be discussed in greater detail in the next chapter.

End Results

The methods of science included in this section can be thought of as the culmination of a series of other processes. But while they mark the end of a particular project of scientific inquiry, they may also be part of an ongoing process.

Drawing Conclusions

The process of drawing conclusions—assertions deduced or induced from premises—was discussed in the section on logical reasoning. It is included again here simply to remind the reader that it is a process with an end result.

Making Interpretations

Making interpretations is the process of giving meaning to observed data. Interpretation takes inquiry beyond statements of what was observed to discussions of what the data indicate and how they should or could be viewed. A research report without any interpretation is not complete—it is merely a statement of findings, leaving the reader with a "so-what" feeling. Investigators are responsible for giving meaning to their findings. Although interpretations may in retrospect not be entirely accurate, not as insightful as they could have been, or even an embarrassment, these possible consequences do not absolve the investigator from the obligation of making interpretations.

Interpretation may take many forms. Three common ones are: (a) clarifying the findings, (b) outlining implications relative to effect or consequence, and (c) putting the information gained into some broader context. It is important not to confuse interpretation with making judgments.

Making Judgments

Making judgments is the process of giving a reasoned

opinion regarding the adequacy, usefulness, importance, or value of something. Terms such as good, bad, valuable, of little worth, accepted, rejected, useful, and not useful are all expressions of judgment.

Judgments are often described as being either objective or subjective. (In actuality many are a combination of the two.) *Objective judgments* are based on some accepted standards or criteria against which the phenomena to be judged are found acceptable or wanting. Objective judgment, for example, could be used in assessing a definition, a research proposal, or an example of deductive reasoning. Criteria for assessing adequacy are available for each of these entities. Objective judgment is open to public scrutiny because the standards or criteria used are available to all. *Subjective judgment* is based on personal opinion or experience. The critic's own standards or criteria—whatever they may be—are used. When making a subjective judgment, the critic should state as clearly as possible the standards and criteria being employed as the basis for judgment. At times, however, the standards or criteria may not be entirely on a conscious level and, thus, be difficult to articulate. Subjective judgments do reflect the critic's biases and values, but, in the end, so do all judgments.

Judgment, at least initially, is based on accepted standards or criteria when they exist. This is followed by subjective judgment. Both types of judgment are important in furthering the work of science. Subjective judgment should not be avoided simply because it is "subjective;" there is nothing wrong with this type of judgment when it is made with care and forethought.

Making judgments within the context of one's own work or the work of close colleagues is usually a private, unstressful endeavor. Making judgments that are public is another matter. When individuals act as critics, they reveal something about themselves. Moreover, they expose their own work to assessment by the same standards or criteria they have used. Some people feel there is too much risk in such a position and avoid making public judgments. This contributes to the rather serious lack of public criticism in many of the health professions. Admittedly, there is some risk in speaking out, but the scientific work of a profession moves forward far more quickly in the presence of well-thought-out public judgment.

Facilitation Processes

The remaining methods of science to be discussed are best described as intellectual activities that take place throughout scientific inquiry—for example, while one is formulating questions, analyzing, or defining. In this sense they facilitate the other methods of science.

Trial and Error

Trial and error is a process in which various methods or means are tried and faulty ones are eliminated in order to find an adequate solution or to achieve a desired result or effect. The process may be overt, in that objects are actively manipulated, or it may be covert, manipulation taking place on an intellectual rather than physical level. Trial and error activities are conducted, for example, in trying to find the relationship between two entities and in seeking categories that will further investigation. Trial and error is usually a fairly directed activity with an end product or goal clearly in mind.

The importance of trial and error in scientific inquiry is often not recognized, particularly by those not intimately involved in such inquiry. The association of trial and error with practical inquiry, of which it is a significant part, makes it seem to some as less than scientific. All science—basic and applied, theoretical, laboratory, and clinical—make considerable use of trial and error. It is inherent and endemic in scientific inquiry.

Reflection

Reflection is the process of thinking about, considering, and deliberating about past events, experiences, or thoughts. Although this method of science was mentioned as one of the major methods used in the phenomenological orientation, it is not unique to that orientation; reflection is used in the scientific activities of all disciplines and professions regardless of epistemological orientation. Reflection is said to be most productive when the individual suspends preconceived ideas as much as possible and comes to the process as a naive participant. Reflection may or may not be goal-directed. Any goal tends to be far less precise than in the trial and error process.

Speculation	Speculation is a process of considering and thinking about phenomena that tends to be more future-oriented than reflection. Speculation is like inductive reasoning; however, it goes far beyond what would usually be considered acceptable in an inductive reasoning process. Conclusions are often guesses based on less than sufficient evidence. Speculation has a playful quality in that any number of ideas are entertained, manipulated, and tossed about without concern for all the niceties of logic. Speculation is a free-floating process and far less directed than trial and error. Engaging in speculation is the fantasy time of the scientist.
Intuition	Intuition is a process whereby an idea is perceived independent of any reasoning process. It is direct apprehension, an immediate insight. Intuitive information comes suddenly, often when a person is not attending to whatever problem is in need of solution. Intuition differs from speculation in that the latter involves a conscious attempt to solve a problem, however circuitous the route. Intuition is not a conscious process. Intuition may occur during speculation, but there is a strong sense on the part of the person that the intuitive information comes from somewhere else. While we are able to follow—at times with some difficulty—the line of thinking during the process of speculation, this is not the case with intuition. We can only trace the chain backwards to discern where the idea *might* have come from, but such retrospective consideration tells us little about the intuitive process. We are frequently unable to identify the origin of an idea gained through intuition. Intuition is not a voluntary process. Time cannot be set aside for such an activity, nor can it be encouraged or shared. Rather, it happens. The only advice that can be given to the young scientist is: "step away from the problem and stop thinking about it; something will come to you."

Intuitive information, as well as that which is gained through reflection and speculation, must eventually be subjected to observation and logical reasoning if one is to have any degree of confidence in the new information.

In conclusion, there are many methods used in the pursuit of scientific knowledge. Each method is important both alone and as it interacts with and enhances other methods. By combining the various methods of science, the fund of knowledge of the human community continues to grow in breadth and depth.

8. *Theory and Its Development*

U nderstanding theory—its characteristics, how it is developed, refined, and tested—is fundamental to formulating adequate sets of guidelines for practice. Information here is presented from the perspective of preparation for applied scientific inquiry, and, thus, some aspects of theory are emphasized over others.

The Characteristics of Theory

This section is concerned with the definition of theory; its structural components—concepts, definitions, and postulates; and the dimensions of theory relative to scope, focus, and process (Broudy, Ennis, & Krimerman, 1973; Hardy, 1973; Kerlinger, 1986; Marx & Cronan-Hillix, 1987; Popper, 1968; Singleton, Straits, Straits, & McAllister, 1988; Vockell, 1983).

Definition of Theory

Theory is an abstract description of a circumscribed set of physical phenomena that delineates the characteristics of the phenomena contained therein and their relationship to each other. Most of the terms in this definition have been discussed previously. However, two may need some clarification. "Abstract description" refers to concern for categories of phenomena, not individual persons, objects, or events. "Circumscribed set of..." refers to what phenomena are and are not addressed in any particular theory. All theories have prescribed boundaries. Only the phenomena within these boundaries—and all of the phenomena therein—are of concern in a given theory.

To understand theory, it is helpful to know what a theory is not. First, a theory is not a single postulate—the relationship between two or more concepts.

Rather, a theory is made up of multiple postulates organized into an integrated whole. A single postulate may be either part of a theory or a piece of empirical data not yet integrated into a theoretical system, but it is not a theory.

A theory is not a discussion of a particular phenomena, sometimes referred to as a "review of the literature." In such a discussion, information from many sources may be brought together for some purpose—for example, to describe how the phenomena have been studied or to identify what is known and not known about the phenomena. Such a discussion may be useful, but it is not a theory.

A theory is not information that is directly used. It is not a description of how to do something or of when or where something ought to be done. For example, a description of how to minimize the formation of excessive scar tissue is not a theory. Such a description may be based on theory or on experience; it may be a partially or fully formed set of guidelines for practice, but it is not a theory. Theories are descriptive only. They exist separate from their use and provide no suggestion for application.

In order to be a theory, an abstract description of phenomena must have the potential to be tested. It must be stated in such a way that the proposed relationship between phenomena is amenable to assessment when adequate tools are available. This is one reason that history is not considered a scientific discipline. Historians are unable to test proposed relationships between events because the phenomena in question no longer exist.

Finally, the question of whether something is or is not a theory has nothing to do with the extent to which it has been tested. Moreover, it is not related to a theory's degree of *validity*—the extent to which a theory allows for accurate prediction about the phenomena addressed. Einstein's general theory of relativity is a theory—both before and after it was tested. And although Needham's theory of spontaneous generation has been demonstrated to be invalid (Hellemans & Bunch, 1988), such a demonstration in no way implies the Needham had not developed a theory or that "spontaneous generation" is no longer a theory.

Like Gertrude Stein's rose, a theory is a theory is a theory. A theory depends upon the phenomena it deals with, its ability to be tested, and its structure.

Structure

The structure of a theory refers to its constituent parts and their arrangement. It is the same regardless of the phenomena addressed. For instance, the general theory of relativity and the theory of spontaneous generation deal with very different phenomena, yet their structure is the same. Similarly, there are many theories of learning, but they all have the same structure. The content of theories varies dramatically; the structure does not.

The components of theory are (a) concepts, (b) definitions, and (c) postulates. In a structurally sound theory, each concept is adequately defined, and the relationships (postulates) of each concept to all others are described. A theory is considered structurally unsound when some concepts are not defined or are inadequately defined, and/or the relationships between some concepts are not stated or not clearly stated. This is illustrated in Figure 4. Theory A represents a structurally sound theory: the circles being concepts, the boxes enclosing the circles adequate definitions, and the solid lines postulates. Theory B illustrates a poorly structured theory. The concept on the left is not defined, the upper right concept inadequately defined. The relationship between some concepts are not stated (no connecting line) or are not clearly stated (dotted line).

Theories in the process of being developed tend to be poorly structured, whereas fully developed theories tend to have a more adequate structure. Theories with a fairly high degree of validity are likely to be more adequately structured than theories with a lesser degree of validity. The relationship between the structural adequacy of a theory and its degree of validity is not necessarily linear, however. One can make up a structurally sound nonsense theory, and a totally invalid theory may be perfectly structured.

Concepts

A concept is an abstract category delineated by specified characteristics. A concept may have only one characteristic, as in the concept "red"—the effect of light with a wavelength of between 610 and 708 nanometers—or it may include multiple characteristics, as in

Figure 4. Structures of theories: complete, incomplete, and with superordinate/subordinate concepts.

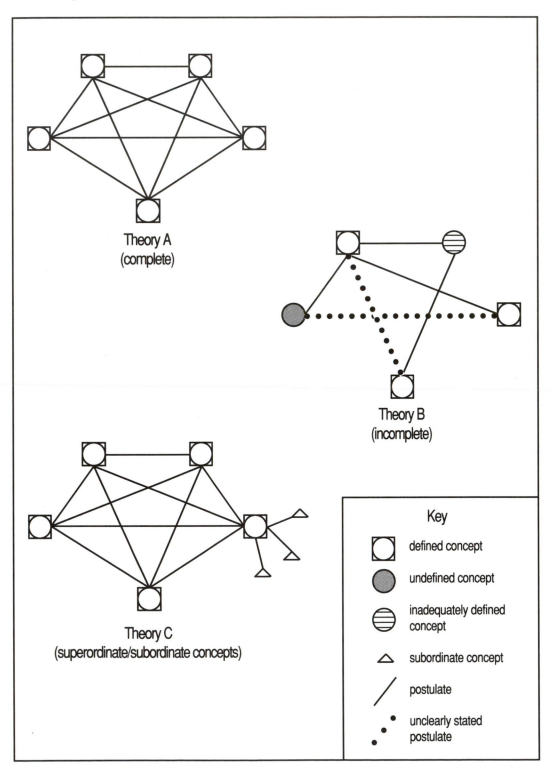

Theory A
(complete)

Theory B
(incomplete)

Theory C
(superordinate/subordinate concepts)

Key

☐ defined concept

⬤ undefined concept

⊜ inadequately defined concept

△ subordinate concept

╱ postulate

⋰ unclearly stated postulate

"porcelain"—a strong, vitreous, translucent ceramic material, biscuit-fired at a low temperature and glost-fired at a very high temperature (Flexner & Hauck, 1987). The number of characteristics is irrelevant; what is relevant is that they are clearly stated.

In order to be shared among people, a concept must have a label—a word, phrase, or sign by which it is known. Concept labels are important for it is through them that we are able to communicate about concepts. A label serves only as the insignia of a concept and should never be mistaken for the concept it denotes. A label has no meaning in and of itself. For example, "pencil" is the label for a category of objects characterized as being, "a slender tube of wood, metal, plastic, etc., containing a core or strip of graphite, a solid coloring material, or the like, used for writing or drawing" (Flexner & Hauck, 1987, p. 1432). Objects that meet this criteria may be called "pencils," but the label is not the concrete entity; it is only the agreed-upon language used to denote a category.

The originator of a concept may select any label for it, but, by the conventions of science, a label should:

1. Not denote a concept in common use in the discipline or profession or in related disciplines or professions.

2. Be dissimilar to labels used in the conceptual system (e.g., theory, taxonomy, or set of guidelines for practice) in which the concept is, or is likely to be, included.

3. Be unlike the labels of somewhat similar concepts used in other conceptual systems.

4. Be neutral in connotation in the major international languages.

Concepts can be categorized in a number of ways. For example, a distinction is made between simple concepts and constructs. A *simple concept* is a category whose characteristics are readily observable because of their visual, tangible qualities—for example, paper clip, lamp shade, automobile, and book. These categories can be described verbally or represented pictorially. *Constructs*, on the other hand, have less tangible characteristics and cannot be directly observed. Examples include temperature, intelligence, need, and learning. Constructs can ultimately only be described through reference to some sort of stimulus-response sequence. Use of an intervening device may also be necessary. For example, learning is said to have occurred when information (stimulus) is presented to a student and, subsequently, the student responds (response) correctly to test questions (intervening device).

Variables are concepts that are defined in such a way that they can be counted or measured. Both simple concepts and constructs may be variables or may be redefined in such a way as to become variables. Thus, the difference between simple concepts/constructs and variables is not in the phenomena they categorize but in the way the category is defined. Quantitative research requires the use of variables; that is, in order to use a quantitative research design, concepts must be defined in such a way that they can be counted or measured. Qualitative research designs do not have such a requirement.

Concepts may be described as being *superordinate* to, *subordinate* to, or *on the same level* with other concepts. The term "conceptual levels" is used to identify this way of ordering concepts. Whether a given concept is superordinate or subordinate is dependent on the other concepts to which it is compared. "Mammal" is superordinate to "whale" but is subordinate to "vertebrate." Concepts on the same level have a common, superordinate concept without any intermediate superordinate concepts. Thus, "whale" and "dolphin" are on the same conceptual level, cetacean being the common superordinate concept. "Whale" and "vertebrate" are not on the same conceptual level because there are several conceptual levels between the subkingdom Metazoa, of which "vertebrate" is immediately subordinate, and "whale."

Specification of conceptual levels is an important organizational component of theory. In Figure 4, the concepts of Theories A and B are on the same conceptual level. Theory C illustrates a difference in conceptual levels. The concept at the far right is on the same level as all or the other concepts, but has three subordinate concepts. This cluster, for example, could have the superordinate concept of "defense mechanisms"; with "projection," "rationalization," and "denial" being the three subordinate concepts. A theory with a concept having only one subordinate concept is not well-structured. As the rules of outlining an essay state: "if there is an A. 1, there must be an A. 2." The phenomena categorized by the single superordinate-subordinate relationship need to be reconceptualized to form a single concept or two concepts on the same level.

Definitions

An adequate definition is a statement that identifies the essential characteristics and fixes the boundaries of a given concept. A definition allows people other than the originator to identify what phenomena are included in the designated category. An adequate definition has specific characteristics and structure:

1. Label of the concept to be defined.

2. Immediate superordinate category to which the concept belongs. Thus, the beginning of the definition of whale should be "is a cetacean." It should not be "is a mammal" because mammal is not the next highest level category.

3. Specific characteristics distinguishing the concept from any other categories included under the previously stated, immediate, superordinate category. Thus, an adequate definition of "whale" would differentiate it from all other categories of animals included in the order Cetacea, such as dolphins and porpoises.

Extraneous characteristics that do not contribute to differentiating one concept from another are not included in an adequate definition for two reasons: (a) nonessential characteristics tend to confuse rather than clarify, often limiting or expanding the category unintentionally; and (b) science has a "rule of parsimony"— that is, to be sparing, concise, and frugal, with nothing in excess. This rule applies to definitions as well as to theories and sets of guidelines for practice.

The following definition illustrates these points: A ladder is a structure consisting of two side pieces between which a series of bars (or rungs) are set at suitable distance forming a means of climbing up and down. "Ladder" is the concept label, "structure" the immediate superordinate category. The remaining portion of the definition specifies the characteristics differentiating ladder from any other structure. Extraneous characteristics, such as material used in construction, height, and whether ladders are free-standing or in need of support, are not included.

There are six kinds of definitions: functional, descriptive, abstract, operational, by example, and circular. (These types are not on the same conceptual level, however.) A *functional definition* describes a concept relative to the action, activity, or purpose of the phenomena that constitute the category. An example is, "intelligence is a cognitive capacity that allows individuals to undertake activities characterized by difficulty, complexity, abstractness, and adaptiveness to a goal."

A *descriptive definition* depicts, in words or pictorial form, what the phenomena look like. The definition of a ladder is primarily a descriptive definition.

An *abstract definition* describes a concept without reference to specific objects, actual instances, practical considerations, or application. Using this type of definition, intelligence is "a cognitive capacity that consists of an individual's total repertoire of those problem-solving and cognitive-discriminate responses that are usual and expected at any given age level and in the larger population unit to which the individual belongs." The term "abstract definition" is also used to denote any definition that is not an operational definition. With this delineation, the functional definition of intelligence would also be considered an abstract definition.

An *operational definition* describes a concept in such a way that it can be measured or counted in some manner. One operational definition of intelligence is: "the total score an individual receives on the Stanford-Binet intelligence test." The descriptive definition of a ladder is also considered to be an operational definition in that it enables one to point to what is a ladder; it allows the phenomena to be counted. Functional definitions may also be operational, as in a "forester is a person having responsibility for maintaining a forest." One can count those individuals responsible for a forest.

Some concepts are more easily described by one

kind of definition than another. Simple concepts typically have functional or descriptive definitions and are difficult to define abstractly or without reference to specific objects. Constructs do not lend themselves to descriptive definitions, and may be somewhat difficult to define operationally. Variables always have an operational definition. Most definitions are a combination of the various kinds of definitions just described.

Science avoids two kinds of definitions: definition by example and circular definitions. A *definition by example* describes a concept by giving one or more instances of the phenomena included in the concept—for instance, "assistive devices are such things as built-up handles for eating utensils, grab-bars, and button hooks." The problem with definition by example is that the essential characteristics of the concept are not delineated. Although definitions made only by example are poor scholarship, examples are sometimes used to clarify definitions. However, this should not be done as a substitute for a careful delineation of the essential characteristics.

Circular definitions use the concept to be defined in the definition of the concept. The author facetiously used a circular definition previously: "a theory is a theory is a theory." Another example is "a defense mechanism is a mechanism used to defend oneself against unacceptable thoughts and ideas." Circular definitions are most likely to occur in defining constructs or when the essential characteristics of a concept are unclear to the definer.

In studying theories, one may encounter several problems regarding definitions. Some concepts may simply not be defined. Other concepts may be inadequately defined, with no immediate superordinate category or insufficient characteristics to distinguish the concept from other concepts. A concept may be used extensively prior to its definition, leaving the reader uncertain about exactly what is being denoted. Finally, a concept may be defined in a piecemeal manner throughout the theory. Thus, readers do not know the essential characteristics of the concept until they have almost finished perusing the theory.

Once the definition of a concept is stated and a

label assigned, the definition and label are joined. This is referred to as concept *definition-label consistency*—the condition of retentive coherence between the definition of, and label for, a concept. In other words, the definition and the label remain the same. Definition-label consistency is of particular importance in description of a theory. Lack of consistency leads to difficulty in comprehension at best—to total confusion, at worst. The rules for definition-label consistency are:

1. The same label is used for the defined concept throughout the theory. Use of a term thought to be synonymous with a label or shortening a compound label (without so specifying) is not acceptable. When a phrase is used as a label, the word order should not be changed.

2. The definition of a labeled concept is never used to describe a different concept.

3. The label of a given concept is never used to denote a different concept.

4. Once stated, the definition of a labeled concept is never altered during the description of a theory. Modification by the addition or deletion of characteristics is not acceptable.

A concept can have only one definition. A concept with more than one significantly different definition is in reality two or more different concepts with the same label. Thus, a statement like, "this concept has too many definitions," reflects a misunderstanding of the nature of concept definition-label consistency. The concept does not have too many definitions; the same label is being used to denote too many different concepts. This problem is somewhat more common in professions than in disciplines. People in disciplines tend to more careful about defining and labeling concepts because such care is demanded by their colleagues.

The rules of concept definition-label consistency are not meant to inhibit theory development or refinement. Theories are frequently altered. Over time, superordinate, subordinate, and/or entirely new concepts may be identified, defined, and labeled. The definition of a given concept may be refined. A concept may be redefined, changing its essential characteristics, or it may be relabeled.

It is not unusual to read a description of a theory one day and read a new version of the same theory a few months later. Concepts, definitions, and labels change rather dramatically, which is one reason why the applied scientist should work from the most recent version of a theory.

Postulates

Postulates, the third structural component of theory, state the relationship between two or more concepts. Postulates hold theories together. Without postulates, concepts would be isolated categories with little meaning or purpose. There are several types of postulates, but, as was the case with concepts, they are not all on the same conceptual level. Some types of postulates can be thought of as being in pairs: temporal and spatial, quantitative and qualitative, correlative and causal. These are briefly discussed, as are hierarchial postulates and hypotheses.

Temporal postulates are relational statements that order events in time. Examples include "most people work during the day and sleep at night" and "birds often begin to sing right after it stops raining." Temporal postulates are common in biological and behavioral theories dealing with human growth and development.

Spatial postulates order events and objects in space—for instance, "the Mississippi River flows south" and "the earth rotates around the sun." Spatial postulates are frequently found in descriptive anatomy, geography, and astronomy. Postulates may be a combination of temporal and spatial, as in "at certain latitudes, some types of leaves change color during the fall season."

Quantitative postulates are relational statements that identify or imply frequency or amount—for example, "women are far more likely to become single parents than are men" and "the cost of living is higher in New York City than in Minneapolis." Precise quantitative postulates are more common in theories of the physical sciences than in the biological and social sciences. This may be due to differences in the degree of variation inherent in the phenomena studied by these disciplines. Temporal and spacial postulates are usually quantitative.

Qualitative postulates are statements describing an essential or distinctive characteristic that marks the relationship between phenomena—for instance, "a special tenderness is seen in the interaction between most mothers and their young children." Qualitative postulates are not merely imprecise quantitative postulates. The postulates of many behavioral theories are qualitative, and qualitative research designs are used to test and refine these theories.

Correlative postulates are statements of the degree to which two phenomena co-vary. In a positive correlation, two phenomena vary in the same direction; they increase or decrease together. In a negative correlation, the phenomena vary in the opposite direction; as one increases the other decreases. Correlations are often expressed in numerical terms, such as, "there is a +.85 correlation between the grades students receive on term papers and grades on the final examination." Perfect correlations, +1.00 or -1.00, are rare. Correlations do not imply causality, they only express the degree of the "going-togetherness" of the phenomena. Even though causality may seem plausible because of the nature the phenomena involved and the high degree of correlation, there is always the possibility of the "third factor"—an unknown factor that accounts for the correlation.

Causal postulates are statements that describe a cause and effect relationship between phenomena. That is, one phenomenon is considered to be the agent that produces the effect in the other phenomenon. Two examples are: "water freezes at a temperature of 0 degrees Celsius" and "infection leads to swelling in the involved body part."

Causal postulates are fairly common in theories of the physical sciences. Theories in the biological and behavioral sciences tend to consist primarily of *quasi-causal postulates*—those that describe "causal factors" rather than single cause-and-effect relationships. To illustrate, poliomyelitis does not occur without the presence of one of the polioviruses, but polioviruses may be present without evidence of poliomyelitis. There are other factors that influence the polioviruses–

poliomyelitis relationship. Similarly, serious problems in childhood may or may not lead to difficulty in taking adult roles.

Many postulates in the biological and behavioral sciences are actually correlations. However, applied scientists often treat correlations, particularly when the numbers are high, as if they were causal. For example, a high correlation between smoking and lung cancer is often interpreted as smoking causes lung cancer. High correlations tend to be treated as causal relationships when no other factor can be found that logically or empirically seems to account for the correlative relationship. Treating correlative relationships as causal is risky. It should be done sparingly, with great care, and with full knowledge that one is doing so.

The two other types of postulates to be discussed are hierarchial postulates and hypotheses. *Hierarchial postulates* state the positional relationship between two or more concepts relative to the level of abstraction (the same level, superordinate, or subordinate)—for example, an oil lamp and a candle both provide light (same level) and adverbs are one of the parts of speech (subordinate–superordinate). Hierarchial postulates are sometimes similar to the first part of adequate definitions. However, they should not be mistaken for definitions.

Hypotheses are postulates developed for the purpose of determining the relationship between two or more concepts. From the perspective of quantitative research designs, hypotheses are postulates with operationally defined concepts. An example of such an hypothesis is "between 18 and 55 years of age, there is a negative correlation between age at last birthday and visual acuity as measured by an eye chart held approximately 14 inches from the eyes." When qualitative research designs are used, the concepts in an hypothesis are not operationally defined.

In summary, the structural components of theory are concepts, the definitions of concepts, and postulates. These components are the same regardless of the phenomena addressed or the validity of the theory.

Dimensions

In addition to structure, theories can be viewed relative to scope, focus, and process. These dimensions are important in applied Type I inquiry when considering the potential of a given theory for use in a set of guidelines for practice.

The scope of a theory refers to the extent of its boundaries and the breadth of the phenomena addressed in the theory. Although the scope of theories is a continuum, Merton (1968) has marked three points, identifying theories as grand, middle range, and "abstract empiricism."

Grand theories, also referred to as comprehensive theories, are global in nature with wide boundaries, encompassing a broad range of phenomena. Concepts tend to be open-ended, all-inclusive, and highly abstract. Examples of grand theories are psychoanalytic theory and the "theory of everything" of physics. Grand theories are sometimes criticized for trying to explain all things, while explaining nothing. They are very difficult to test. The use of grand theories in applied Type I scientific inquiry is often frustrating and not very successful. They are just too amorphous to work with.

Middle-range theories, as the name implies, are more limited in scope, addressing only small aspects of the physical universe. Concepts tend to be specifically defined and easily related to phenomena. Middle-range theories usually have more concepts than grand theories because phenomena are grouped into more discrete and smaller categories. They are fairly easy to test due to the specificity of concepts. Middle-range theories are more accurate in terms of description and prediction than are grand theories. Regardless of the discipline of origin, the majority of theories are middle range, which are the most frequently used as the basis for sets of guidelines for practice.

Theories referred to as *abstract empiricism* are narrow in scope, dealing with a very limited range of phenomena. They tend to have fewer concepts then middle-range theories. Theories at the level of abstract empiricism often address phenomena in the here and now—for example, the behavior of students in a particular course in fall, 1991. If the exemplary theory were concerned with the behavior of students in all graduate courses, it would be a middle-range theory. Abstract empiricist theories may address such limited and esoteric phenomena that they are not considered particularly relevant to the general goal of science— a theory about coffee consumption among firefighters in Philadelphia, for example.

While theories at the level of abstract empiricism may serve as the nucleus for the development of middle-range theories, they are usually not considered to be of much worth. They may be used in applied scientific inquiry, but usually only in the absence of other more suitable theories or empirical data.

Focus

Focus here refers to the biological-behavioral dimension of theories. This dimension is a continuum along which theories may be primarily biological, a mixture of biological and behavioral, or primarily behavioral.

Biological theories describe the structures and processes of the body with no attempt to relate them to nonreflexive behavior. They are usually made up primarily of simple concepts, although some constructs may be used relative to process.

Behavioral theories describe nonreflexive behavior without recourse to biological phenomena. Some behavioral theories consist primarily of simple concepts like, for example, theories describing milestones in the motor development of a child. Others make considerable use of constructs. This is evident in personality theories, for example, which use such constructs as needs, drives, motivation, and so forth.

Mixed biological-behavioral theories address the relationship between biological structures and processes and nonreflexive behavior. Relationships tend to be expressed as quasi-causal and unidirectional. In other words, biological phenomena are viewed as being the cause of an effect, as in "increased rigidity of the lens of the eye leads to presbyopia," not the reverse. Or, conversely, behavior is described as the cause of specific biological changes, as in "exercise leads to an increase in muscle size."

Mixed biological-behavioral theories are more problematic than either strictly biological or behavioral theories when developing sets of guidelines for practice. They tend to be less valid either because they have not been adequately studied or because of the high degree of variability in the phenomena. This is particularly true in theories regarding relationships between the central nervous system and cognitive and psychological processes.

Another problem is more social in nature. Some health professions tend to prefer mixed biological-behavioral theories because they seem more sophisticated, adding stature to the profession. Mixed theories, particularly those with a neurological component, are sometimes used as the basis for sets of guidelines for practice when behavioral theories would seem to provide a better, more valid foundation. For example, while there is considerable evidence for the biological origin of learning disabilities and schizophrenia, it is questionable whether mixed theories addressing these phenomena are suitable as the foundation for sets of guidelines concerned with habilitation/rehabilitation where focus is primarily on change in behavior rather than change in neurological status.

Mixed biological-behavioral theories *may* be useful for sets of guidelines for practice. But care must be taken in selecting and extrapolating from such theories. One should apply *Occam's razor*, one of the guiding principles of science taken from the work of 14th century English philosopher William Occam: when several explanations of a phenomenon are offered, the simplest should be taken.

Process

Process refers to the extent to which theories are concerned with change. Theories can be viewed relative to process on a continuum of dynamic to static. *Dynamic theories* address such issues as how change takes place, how it is inhibited or maintained, and how the condition of homeostasis is sustained. *Static theories*, on the other hand, describe phenomena as if they were fixed or in terms of increments of change without describing how change occurs. Many theories have both dynamic and descriptive components.

Kinesiology is an example of a theory at the dynamic end of the process continuum, whereas descriptive human anatomy is an example of a theory at the static end of the continua. The various theories of learning are also examples of dynamic theories. Theories dealing with human development are usually thought of as dynamic, yet many of them are essentially static because they describe various stages of development but say little about how the individual moves from one stage to the next, other than by describing unspecified interaction in an ill-defined environment. This is illustrated in theories regarding gross motor development and the various stages of children's play.

Dynamic theories are essential in formulating sets of guidelines for practice in most health professions. Intervention is concerned with change itself, inhibiting unwanted change, and maintaining change—only dynamic theories can provide theoretical support for such activities. Static theories are also important as they are used to delineate and describe the area of human function of concern in sets of guidelines for practice. However, static theories alone cannot support a set of guidelines.

In conclusion, theories are the structures used for organizing knowledge derived from basic scientific inquiry. They have a variety of characteristics that, when understood, facilitate formulation of sets of guidelines for practice. Prior to moving on to that topic however, two other areas must be explored: (a) taxonomies and (b) the developing, testing, and, refining of theories. Taxonomies are discussed first because they are sometimes a precursor to theory development.

Taxonomies

A taxonomy is a conceptual system that orders phenomena into different categories and sometimes according to various levels of abstraction. Examples include the periodic table of elements; the classification of animals and plants into phylum, class, order, and so forth; and the epistemological orientations to practice outlined in Chapter 2. Almost all phenomena can be arranged in a systematic manner. Taxonomies bring organization to what appear to be highly disparate and variable phenomena.

Taxonomies are not theories. Like theories, they describe and order phenomena, but they do not allow for making predictions about phenomena. The formation of a taxonomy or taxonomies is often the first activity undertaken by a new field of scientific inquiry. In addition to sometimes being the initial step in theory development, taxonomies are briefly discussed here for two other reasons. First, they are frequently found in basic and applied science literature. Second, because taxonomies should not be mistaken for theories, information about taxonomies is presented to minimize any confusion.

There is no absolute scheme of classification for any given set of phenomena. Categories are not inherent in phenomena, nor in the way phenomena are ordered. The areas of human function included in a particular profession's domain of concern can be and have been classified in many different ways.

The purpose for which a taxonomy is developed is important because it strongly influences the formation of categories. Categories are selected to emphasize the properties of the phenomena of concern to the developer/consumer. The essential question in assessing a taxonomy is: "Does it work for the purpose intended?" For example, television programs may be categorized by time of day presented, types of content, suitability for a particular audience, and so forth. The usefulness of the categories is dependent on the purpose for which the taxonomy is developed. In developing a taxonomy, as in any process of categorizing, the selected distinctive features of each category are specified, and other features, considered unimportant, are excluded or ignored. If one were developing a taxonomy of television programs for the purpose of elucidating types of content, the time of day the programs are aired would not be relevant.

There are several types of taxonomies, but only the major ones will be briefly described here. As taxonomies are so influenced by their purpose, many of them are quite idiosyncratic. A given taxonomy may be like one of the types to be described, a combination of two or more of the types, or in no way resemble any of them. The types are presented according to degree of complexity.

Cluster taxonomies consist of broad groupings based on similarity or contiguity of phenomena. Cluster taxonomies based on similarities may use one or several characteristics for identifying categories. An example of the former is categorizing animals by what they eat: carnivorous, herbivorous, and omnivorous. An example of the latter are the multiple characteristics used to identify various types of dessert: cake, pie, pudding, and so forth. Cluster taxonomies based on contiguity group phenomena that are close together in some way, for instance, time (Cenozoic, Mesozoic, Paleozoic and Precambrian) or place (North America, Middle America and South America).

Pragmatic taxonomies consist of categories developed without concern for the niceties of any one scheme of organization, criteria, or conceptual levels. Such taxonomies violate all of the usual rules of systematic classification. Nevertheless, when they serve the purpose for which they were created, such taxonomies are considered quite acceptable. A good example of a pragmatic taxonomy is the grouping of diagnostic categories in the *Diagnostic and Statistical Manual of Mental Disorders III-R* (American Psychiatric Association, 1987). One grouping is based on age of onset, another on the course of conditions, and others on observable behavior, precipitating events, and systems affected. Areas of specialization as delineated by many health professions often take the form of a pragmatic taxonomies.

Equivalency taxonomies consist of categories on the same level with no implication of superordination or subordination relative to value, amount, time, or any other criteria. The social roles of concern for occupational therapists—involvement in self-care, family, work, and play/recreation—are an example of an equivalency taxonomy because none of these roles is considered to be more important than the others. The various parts of speech in grammar are also organized in an equivalency taxonomy.

Rank order taxonomies consist of categories arranged in a graded fashion along one dimension. Categories are considered superordinate or subordinate to each other based on specific criteria. Examples include academic levels—grade school, high school, college, graduate school—and military ranks.

Hierarchical taxonomies consist of categories at different levels of abstraction in which all categories, except the lowest, include two or more subordinate categories. Such taxonomies are often presented in the form of a rough pyramid—for instance, genealogical trees and the arrangement of the Indo-European languages into families, subfamilies, dialects, and subdialects. Some taxonomies are hierarchical-like in that they do not strictly adhere to all of the criteria described in the definition. The organizational charts of some businesses are hierarchical-like in that a few positions do not fall neatly into the typical pyramid. A supervisor of art acquisitions, for instance, might report directly to the company president and be outside of the usual chain of communication.

The relationship between the categories of a taxonomy may or may not be relevant, depending on the purpose of the taxonomy. They are relevant, for example, in a hierarchical taxonomy, but not in a cluster taxonomy. Whatever they may be, relationships between categories are never causal or correlative.

Taxonomies strongly influence the way we view phenomena. A taxonomy may take on such a sense of reality that one comes to believe the phenomena are truly organized in that manner and can be ordered in no other way. For example, we tend to believe there really are animal phyla and classes. Viewing phenomena through the filter of a taxonomy leads to some degree of bias, inhibiting alternative ways of perceiving phenomena.

Developing, Refining, and Testing Theory

Developing, refining, and testing any theory are usually long-term processes. One person may take primary responsibility, or many people, sometimes distant in time and place, may participate. Basic scientific inquiry is a complex process consisting of many steps and is rarely a smooth journey from beginning to end; it involves fits and starts, false paths, circling back, wasted time, and occasionally being completely lost. Perseverance is requisite.[1]

From one perspective, formulating a theory may begin anywhere on the continuum of the field/laboratory to the ivory tower. The process usually involves moving back and forth along the continuum. Theory

---

[1] The following description draws upon the work of Kerlinger, (1986), Marx & Cronan-Hillix (1987), Phillips (1987), Popper (1968), Regis (1987), Singleton, Straits, Straits, & McAllister (1988) and Vockell (1983).

Figure 5. "From the field or laboratory": pictorial representation of beginning theory development and refinement in the field or laboratory.

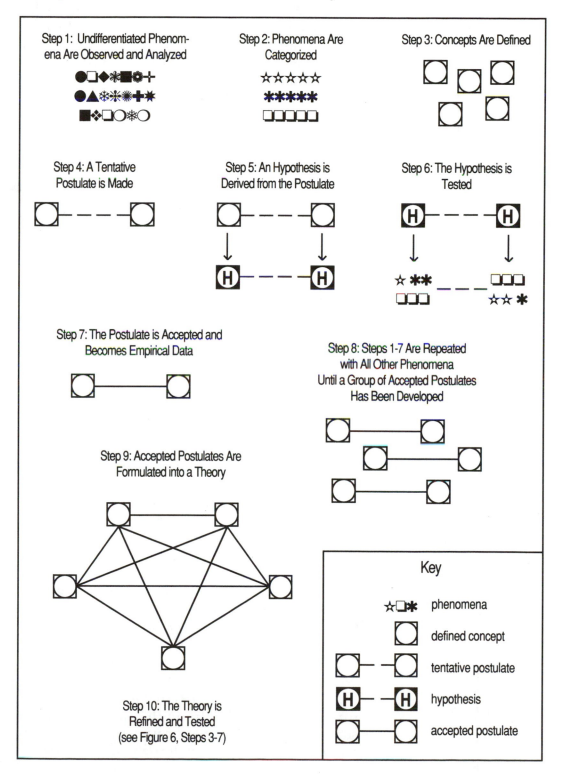

development is first outlined here as it begins in the field/laboratory, followed by theory development from the other end of the continuum, the ivory tower. The latter includes a description of how the theory is tested to assess its degree of validity—that is, the extent to which it leads to accurate predictions about the phenomena addressed. Special attention is not given to theory refinement because this occurs simultaneously with, and is an intimate part of, development and testing. The third part of this section is concerned with some issues related to validity of theories.

Developing, refining, and testing theory is described here within the context of quantitative research designs because they, unlike qualitative designs, use variables and hypotheses.

From the Field or Laboratory

"From the field or laboratory" refers to theory development that begins with direct involvement in undifferentiated, uncategorized phenomena. The scientist's task is to describe and order the phenomena to determine relationships among them, and to develop valid theory. Figure 5 illustrates the steps involved in completing the task.

Step 1   At this stage there is a jumble of undifferentiated phenomena, seemingly quite uniform perhaps or hopelessly diverse. The scientist studies the phenomena: observes, analyzes, speculates, and reasons.

Step 2   Particular elements of the phenomena are recognized, and at least some of their identifying characteristics are deciphered; classification has begun. Provisional categories are developed. Categories may be quite broad at first, becoming more refined later in the process. On the other hand, categories may be initially too narrow. In the process of theory development, phenomena thought at first to be dissimilar may be found to be sufficiently similar to be combined into one category. Categories are labeled primarily for the purpose of communication; more permanent labels may be selected later. At least two categories must be formed for theory development to continue.

Step 3   The categories—now referred to as concepts—are formally defined although the immediate, superordinate concept may be vague or simply not be included. The adequacy of the definitions is assessed through comparison to the phenomena. The question asked is, "Do these definitions allow for the inclusion of all the desired phenomena and the exclusion of all other phenomena?" One or more taxonomies may be developed at this point.

Step 4 As the result of further observation, speculation, and so forth, a relationship—a tentative postulate—between two concepts is proposed.

Step 5 Does the proposed postulate reflect the actual relationship of the phenomena in question? Postulates cannot be tested directly; they must be assessed indirectly by testing hypotheses. Thus, an hypothesis is deduced from the postulate. This process includes formulating operational definitions for the concepts and making them into variables. The form of the hypothesis—the language in which it is stated—is dependent on the type of relationship being tested and the particular research design being employed.

Step 6 The hypothesis is tested by designing a situation in which the proposed relationship between the phenomena can be observed in a controlled manner. The findings are analyzed, synthesized, and interpreted in order to see whether they support the hypothesis. An investigator is rarely comfortable in stating whether a postulate is supported by the findings based on the testing of only one hypothesis. Thus, additional hypotheses are usually deduced from the postulate and tested. In testing hypotheses, the relationship between concepts is assessed, not the concepts themselves or their definitions. However, when a proposed relationship is not found, the concepts may be reexamined to see if there may be a problem with the way in which the phenomena have been categorized.

Step 7 When the investigator is satisfied with the results derived from testing various hypotheses deduced from the postulate, the postulate is considered "accepted" and becomes a piece of empirical data.

Step 8 At this point only two elements of the phenomena have been considered. The process of theory development continues by repeating Steps 1 through 7 until all elements of the phenomena have been accounted for. Over time, a variety of tentative postulates are formulated, hypotheses are deduced, and all are tested. When found to accurately reflect the phenomena, the postu-

Figure 6. "From the ivory tower": pictorial representation of beginning theory development, refinement, and testing in the ivory tower.

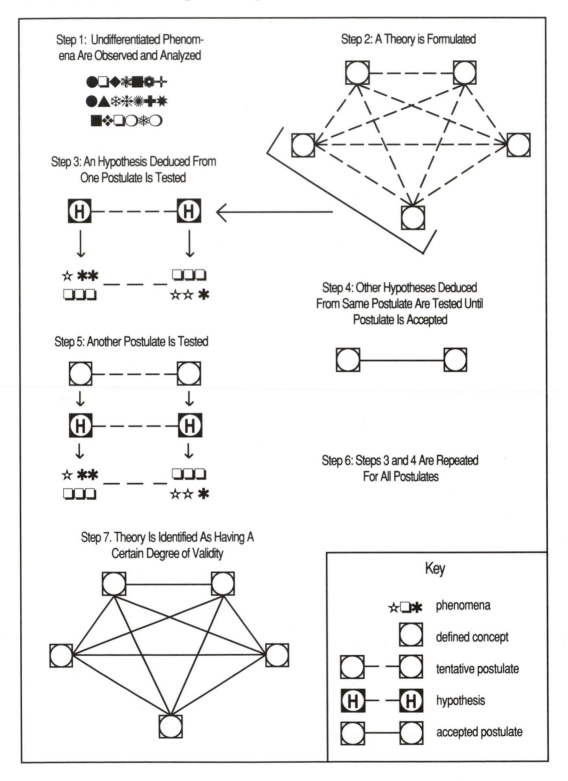

Applied Scientific Inquiry in the Health Professions

lates enter the realm of empirical data, creating considerable knowledge about the phenomena but no theory.

Step 9   All the empirical data generated in Steps 1 through 7 are synthesized and integrated into the formal structure of a theory. All the pieces of the puzzle are set into place.

Step 10   Although many of the postulates of the theory have been tested, the theory itself must now be tested. This is done for two reasons: (a) new, untested postulates were probably formed to enable the empirical data to be integrated into the formal structure of a theory, and (b) articulation of the theory may have changed some of the previously tested postulates. Through testing, the theory is further refined.

An analogy may clarify why theories developed in the above manner need to be tested: When one sees only the parts of an unassembled toy, neither the parts nor the whole is well understood. Once assembled, the parts and purpose of each part make sense and the whole becomes better known. Then, in order to find out whether it works, the whole must first be tried out and perhaps fine-tuned. The same is true of a theory; it must be tested and refined. When Step 10 is complete and all of the empirical data are integrated into the formal structure of a theory, the theory is ready for final testing and, if necessary, revision. This process is the same as Steps 3 through 7 of ivory tower theory development, as described in the next section.

From the Ivory Tower   "From the ivory tower" refers to theory development, refinement, and testing that begins with contemplation of an undifferentiated collection of phenomena from a distance. The task of the scientist is to develop a theory with no immediate direct involvement with the phenomena at this point. Later, with direct involvement with the phenomena, the originator of the theory or other scientists are concerned with determining the validity of the theory. Figure 6 illustrates the steps involved.

Step 1   This step is quite similar to the first step of the field or laboratory approach. There is observation, speculation, analysis, and probably a good deal of reflection.

Step 2   A theory is formulated. It is not clear what specific intellectual processes and steps are involved; intuition may play a part. In any event, a reaonable-looking theory is there. Now, the task of the scientist is to assess the theory's degree of validity. Refinement of the theory is also likely to be necessary.

Step 3   Theories cannot be tested as a whole; rather, they are tested postulate by postulate. And since postulates cannot be tested directly, testing a theory begins by selecting one postulate, deducing an hypothesis from that postulate, and testing the hypothesis using a research design appropriate to the form and language of the hypothesis. For example, one postulate of a theory about development of group interaction skills is: "Children between the ages of 2 and 4 years have the ability to engage in a project group" (Mosey, 1986). (A "project group" is characterized by participants' involvement with others in a short-term task that requires some shared interaction, cooperation, and competition.) From this postulate, an hypothesis could be derived: "At least 75% of the 3-year-old children in day care center X will actively participate (not leave) in a seven-person circle game for 10 minutes." To test this hypothesis, a survey research design could be used that simply required counting the number of children who did not leave the circle game during the 10-minute period. After analysis, synthesis, and interpretation of the findings, a judgment is made as to whether the findings support the hypothesis.

Step 4   As has been mentioned, postulates are generally not viewed as accurately reflecting the phenomena in question on the basis of testing only one deduced hypothesis. Thus, several related hypotheses are derived from the given postulate and tested prior to accepting the postulate. How much testing is needed cannot be stated in any precise way; hypotheses continue to be tested until a scientist believes—and/or there is general recognition by the scientific community—that the postulate is sufficiently accurate that no further testing is required at this time.

The postulates of some theories have not been subjected to sufficient basic scientific inquiry to warrant general acceptance—for example, the relationship between estrogen and breast cancer. Other postulates have been subjected to excessive inquiry; the

Applied Scientific Inquiry in the Health Professions

relationship between positive reinforcement and change in behavior is one example.

Step 5   Another postulate from the theory is selected for study; various hypotheses are deduced and tested.

Step 6   Steps 3 and 4 are repeated relative to each postulate of the theory. Only after completion of this process are statements about the validity of a theory as a whole able to be made with any confidence.

Step 7   The testing of the theory is now complete, and thus its degree of validity has been determined. With a known degree of validity, the theory can be knowledgeably used—or not used—as the basis for sets of guidelines for practice.

Issues Related to Validity   Validity refers to the accuracy with which a theory describes, and allows for accurate prediction about, the phenomena addressed. A theory may be considered invalid—that is, it does not accurately reflect the phenomena of concern. However, when a theory is said to be valid, the validity is usually expressed as relative, a matter of degree. For example, it may be said that "theory X is the most valid currently available" or "theory X is more valid than theory Y."

As mentioned in Chapter 6, theories are never considered "true." The search for truth is not part of the business of science, for science is forever fallible. Basic science is concerned with understanding the physical universe by finding out more about it. Feynman (1985) used the analogy of peeling an onion, understanding the universe layer by layer; at each layer our comprehension is different. But he also acknowledged that the analogy breaks down because the onion of the physical universe is unlikely to ever be completely peeled.

A thoughtful scientist knows the theory he or she developed today will probably be supplanted by a more valid theory—tomorrow, next year, or sometime in the more distant future. In some cases a theory is substantially revised leading to a greater degree of validity. At other times, a theory is not simply revised; it is replaced by an entirely new theory. The new theory is considered to be more valid and, in fact, demonstrates the invalidity of the old theory. For example, the theory of immutable species was made invalid as a result of the development and testing of the theory of biological evolution.

Theories can be described as having *face validity* and/or empirical validity. Face validity refers to how plausible a theory seems based on what is already known about the phenomena from personal experience, and common sense. Assessing face validity is often the first step in evaluating a theory. It is the only measure of validity available when a theory has not yet been tested or cannot be tested due to the lack of adequate research tools. When necessary, such theories are used in applied scientific inquiry, albeit with a good deal of caution. Face validity, however, may be a poor predictor of empirical validity. Many theories demonstrated to have a high degree of empirical validity fly in the face of experience and common sense. Experience and common sense tell us the earth is flat, for instance.

Empirical validity refers to the extent to which the findings of basic scientific inquiry support a theory. Documentation of empirical support for a given theory may not be found all in one place or in a concise manner; one must often search for this information. The factors examined in assessing the empirical validity of a theory are: (a) the extent of inquiry, (b) the relationship between the hypotheses tested and the postulates of the theory, (c) the types of research designs used, (d) the adequacy of designs relative to the theory being tested, (e) the data gathered, (f) the manner in which the data were treated, and (g) how findings have been interpreted.

The validity of a theory must be established relative to other theories; therefore, the same information must be gathered regarding other theories that address the same phenomena. Only at this point can an individual make a sound judgment about the empirical validity of a given theory. This last step, comparative analysis, is not taken when there is no other theory that addresses the phenomena of concern, but such a situation is fairly uncommon, at least in the behavioral sciences. Competing theories are theories with relatively equal empirical validity that address the same phenomena. Selection of one rather than another competing theory for use in applied scientific inquiry is based on factors other than validity. These criteria are discussed in Chapter 10.

Sometimes health professions use criteria other than the degree of empirical support in considering use of a theory in a set of guidelines for practice. Practitioners are swayed by the extent to which a theory has been used, in whole or in part, as a basis for a variety of sets of guidelines in different professions. For example, learning theories have been used without any clear idea of their validity. The newness or popularity of a theory can also affect its perceived validity. A theory may suddenly come into vogue; everyone is reportedly using it as the basis for sets of guidelines for practice, but the validity of the theory is not discussed in much detail, if at all. For a time, everyone seemed to be using Piaget's theory of cognitive development, for example.

There are no definitive answers to the questions: "How valid is valid?" or "When is a theory sufficiently valid to use as the foundation for a set of guidelines for practice?" In many cases, it is simply a matter of judgment. Being conservative and taking risks are both part of applied scientific inquiry.

Section IV:
Applied Scientific Inquiry

As has been indicated earlier, there is far less known about applied scientific inquiry than about basic inquiry. Applied inquiry has not been studied in any depth by philosophers of science or by those more immediately involved in the process, and, thus, there are gaps in our understanding.

The first chapter of this section is concerned with defining applied scientific inquiry and describing its relationship to basic inquiry. The use of applied scientific inquiry in formulating—developing, refining, and assessing—sets of guidelines for practice is outlined. Chapter 10 provides a general description of the process, including some observations that pertain to sets of guidelines in all professions. Chapter 11 provides a more detailed discussion of the development of sets of guidelines for practice in occupational therapy.

9. *The Nature of Applied Scientific Inquiry*

Applied scientific inquiry, ill-defined in the literature (if defined at all), seems to have an amorphous nature, leading to uncertainty among the public and scientists alike about what it is. Individuals often confuse basic scientific inquiry with applied inquiry, but fruitful engagement in either basic or applied scientific inquiry can only take place when a scientist is clear as to the nature and purpose of his or her inquiry.

In General

As described in Chapter 1, applied scientific inquiry is a form of investigation that uses the methods of science and either theoretical information or research designs for the purpose of arriving at immediate practical ends. Practical ends means taking some course of action or answering a specific question for the expressed purpose of satisfying human needs. This concern for immediate practical ends—rather than only the desire to know or understand—is one of the characteristics differentiating applied scientific inquiry from basic inquiry.

One of the problems in understanding applied scientific inquiry is its treatment as a single entity or process in the literature—that is, no distinction is made between using theoretical information as the foundation for making or doing something and using research designs to answer practical questions. For example, extrapolating from theories and empirical data to develop a comprehensive exercise program for pre-adolescents and designing, conducting, and interpreting a public opinion poll are both referred to as applied scientific inquiry. Placing these two activites in one category, with no subdivisions, can cause confusion. What applied scientists do to design an exercise program is quite different from what they do to design a public opinion poll. Most importantly, the former requires use of theoretical information, while the latter does not. Thus, to facilitate understanding, applied scientific inquiry is divided in this text into two subcategories—applied Type I inquiry and applied Type II inquiry.

Applied Type I inquiry is the process whereby theories and empirical data are used as the basis for developing sets of guidelines for action. Guidelines for action may be concerned with fabricating technological products (sets of technological guidelines) or with the process of problem identification and resolution with clients (sets of guidelines for practice). Sets of guidelines for practice are the focus here, although at times reference is made to sets of technological guidelines or sets of guidelines for action in general.

Applied Type II inquiry is the process in which the methods of science and research designs are used to answer specific practical questions. Although the questions may vary widely, they are primarily concerned with assessing amount, safety, quality, worth, and effectiveness. Applied Type II inquiry is used in refining and assessing the adequacy of sets of guidelines for practice and in addressing practical questions outside of the context of sets of guidelines for action. In the health professions, these questions are typically concerned with demographics and activities of a profession, practitioners' opinions about various issues, the needs of different client populations, and professional and postprofessional education.

The two types of applied scientific inquiry are used both alone and in conjunction with each other. Applied Type II inquiry, however, is more likely to be used alone than is applied Type I inquiry because when applied Type II inquiry is focused on addressing practical questions—such as determining how many children in the U.S. live in single-parent households—it is unrelated to developing sets of guidelines for action. Conversely, formulating sets of guidelines for practice involves both applied Type I and Type II inquiry. Simply put, applied Type I inquiry is used for developing sets of guidelines for practice; applied Type II inquiry for refining and assessing the adequacy of sets of guidelines for practice. "Assessment of adequacy" means determining the reliability and validity of problem identification and the safety, effectiveness, efficiency, and acceptability to clients of problem resolution.

To illustrate the differences between applied inquiry and basic inquiry and between the two types of applied inquiry, take the example of two groups of investigators testing the effectiveness of insect repellents (Schwartz, 1989). The first group, working in the Everglades, examines many repellents made by pharmaceutical companies as well as home remedies sent to them by the public. Testing is systematized, using accepted and appropriate scientific methods and research designs. Evaluation of effectiveness is based on counting how many insect bites there are on an individual's unprotected leg compared to a leg covered with insect repellent and/or clothing. This is an example of applied Type II inquiry. Meanwhile, in Menlo Park, California, other investigators are taking a different approach, attempting to determine the "molecular interactions of attractants with receptors on mosquitos' antennas" (p. 86). This is an example of basic inquiry. Mosquito repellent developed from theoretical knowledge gained at Menlo Park would involve applied Type I inquiry. The adequacy of this new repellent could then be subjected to applied Type II inquiry back in the Everglades.

Attempts to define and describe applied scientific inquiry have been traditionally couched in terms of comparison with basic inquiry. Until there is greater understanding of applied inquiry, this is a reasonable approach and, to a great extent, is used here. However, four criteria that were used in the past have been identified as inappropriate for distinguishing applied scientific inquiry from basic inquiry: (a) the person doing the inquiry, (b) the setting of the inquiry, (c) "relevance," and (d) sequence in which the inquiry takes place (Broudy, Ennis, & Krimerman, 1973; Carroll, 1968; Downs, 1979; Grove, 1989).

The occupation of the individual engaging in scientific inquiry does not differentiate applied inquiry from basic inquiry (Grove, 1989). On occasion, members of a profession may engage in basic inquiry; members of a discipline in applied inquiry. Change in an individual's typical form of scientific inquiry is seen most often when members of professions and disciplines are working closely together on an urgent project—for instance, creating the atomic bomb or the scientific inquiry associated with AIDS. Those individuals who want to make a change from one form of inquiry to another on a permanent basis tend to seek academic or apprentice education to prepare themselves for such a change.

The setting in which scientific inquiry takes place does not distinguish applied inquiry from basic inquiry (Downs, 1979). Either form of inquiry, and the attendant research involved, may be conducted in a clinical, laboratory, or field setting. Thus, the term "clinical research" should not be used synonymously with "applied research." Basic research may take place in a clinical setting; applied research in a laboratory setting.

Relevance, in the sense of bearing upon resolution of a practical problem, does not differentiate applied inquiry from basic inquiry (Carroll, 1968). Projects using basic scientific inquiry may be specifically designed to provide theoretical information essential to the solution of a practical problem. Such basic inquiry, then, would be very relevant. Applied scientific inquiry is designed to address practical problems, but that does not mean that all findings generated through applied inquiry have immediate relevance.

Some assume that the linear sequence of basic inquiry-to-applied inquiry is inviolable. Although this is a common sequence, it is by no means invariant. Findings from applied inquiry often lead to basic inquiry. "What comes first" is not a good criterion for differentiating between applied and basic inquiry. The various relationships between applied and basic inquiry—including sequence—are discussed in more detail in the last section of this chapter.

Finally, it should be noted that an area of basic scientific inquiry does not become an applied field of study just because some of the theories generated by the area of study have been applied (Broudy, Ennis, & Krimerman, 1973). Similarly, an area of applied scientific inquiry does not become a basic field of study when the findings generated by the area of study have prompted basic scientific inquiry.

Applied Type I Inquiry

Applied Type I inquiry must be differentiated from practical inquiry. Practical inquiry involves observation, reasoning, trial and error, and taking advantage of fortuitous happenings to arrive at practical ends without recourse to systematic use of theoretical information. Conversely, applied Type I inquiry does make use of theoretical information. When practical inquiry is used to develop sets of guidelines for practice, the guidelines are atheoretical. Atheoretical sets of guidelines for action may be subjected to applied Type II inquiry and found to be quite adequate, but they remain atheoretical until a theory or empirical data can be found to support them.

There are four major characteristics that differentiate applied Type I scientific inquiry from basic inquiry: the fundamental question, the goal, the process, and the end product (Ausubel, 1953; Broudy, Ennis, & Krimerman, 1973; Carroll, 1968; Downs, 1979; Feibleman, 1983; Jarvie, 1983, 1986; Kneller, 1978; Merton, 1982; Mosey, 1989; Van Melsen, 1961; Wulff, Pedersen, & Rosenberg, 1986).

The Fundamental Question

In applied Type I inquiry, the fundamental question is: "What theories and empirical data can be used as the foundation for guidelines directed toward dealing with a specific problem?" The investigator is concerned with finding useful theoretical information, not creating it. In basic inquiry, the fundamental question is: "What is the nature of the phenomena?" The individual is concerned only with gaining greater understanding of particular phenomena, not with practical problems.

The Goal

The goal of applied Type I inquiry is to develop theoretically based sets of guidelines for practice that provide adequate direction for dealing with specific problems. This involves using the most valid theoretical information currently available. The goal of basic scientific inquiry is to develop valid theories—those that allow for accurate prediction about the phenomena of concern. The potential application of the theory is not an issue.

Process of Inquiry

The literature does not clearly outline how one actually engages in applied Type I inquiry and develops sets of guidelines for practice—unlike the processes of basic scientific inquiry which are known and well-described. In discussing applied Type I inquiry, some recent authors, referring to Ausubel (1953) and Carroll (1968), identify the process as one of "extrapolation." However, neither Ausubel nor Carroll defined extrapolation, nor did they provide any information about what, if any, steps are involved in the process. Other authors refer to the process as "deduction." For example, Wulff, Pedersen, and Rosenberg (1986) view applied Type I inquiry in medicine as deducing treatment from the descriptions of disease mechanisms developed through basic inquiry. However, on closer reading, these authors and Jarvie (1986) seem to be describing a process of inductive rather than deductive reasoning.

Looking in more detail at the terms used in discussing applied Type I inquiry—to *extrapolate* is "to infer (an unknown) from something that is known" (Flexner & Hauck, 1987, p. 686). *Inference* is a "process of arriving at some conclusion that though it is not logically derivable from the assumed premises, possesses some degree of probability related to the premises" (Flexner & Hauck, 1987, p. 978). *Deductive reasoning* is a logical process wherein the conclusion follows necessarily from the premises on which it is based. On the other hand, *inductive reasoning* is a process wherein conclusions are proposed that go beyond the evidence presented in the premises.

The literature and the above definitions seem to indicate that the process of applied Type I inquiry involves a logical leap from a problem to theoretical information or from theoretical information to a problem. Once this gap has been bridged and a connection made, deductive reasoning seems to play a greater role. Logical reasoning is not the only process in-

Applied Scientific Inquiry in the Health Professions

volved in applied Type I inquiry. All of the methods of science outlined in Chapter 7 are used with none being more or less important. However, reasoning is given a dominant place in the professional literature.

The process of applied Type I inquiry is best described in reports about developing a particular set of guidelines for action. The process does not seem to be all of one piece, nor is it linear. Instead, there appear to be steps that are repeated several times in a circular or spiral-like manner. Five steps are involved:

1. Analysis of a problem.

2. Identification of suitable theories/empirical data.

3. Selection and synthesis of germane postulates to form a theoretical foundation.

4. Deduction from the theoretical foundation of:

   a. Guidelines for fabricating a technological product, or

   b. Guidelines for identifying and resolving a clinical problem.

5. Consideration of internal consistency and completeness of content.

These steps are described in more detail in Chapter 10. For now, it should be noted that applied Type I inquiry can begin with either theoretical information or a problem in need of solution. In other words, steps 1 and 2 may be reversed.

Applied Type I inquiry does not involve the use of research designs. This is troubling to some people because they equate scientific inquiry with research designs and research projects. This misconception only leads to general confusion. Research designs *are* used in applied Type II to refine and assess the adequacy of sets of guidelines for practice, however. The two types of inquiry may be interrelated in formulating a specific set of guidelines for practice, but they should not be confused with each other.

Product of Inquiry Another way of distinguishing between applied Type I scientific inquiry and basic inquiry is by examining their end products, sets of guidelines for practice and theories, respectively. As the characteristics of theories have been discussed, and since sets of guidelines for practice will be discussed in greater depth in the following chapters, the following is stated very briefly. Five categories are used for comparing the products of inquiry:

Source The source of sets of guidelines for practice is theoretical information—theories and empirical data. The source of theory, on the other hand is raw, undifferentiated data.

Purpose The purpose of sets of guidelines for practice is to: (a) transform theories so that they can be applied, (b) link theories to practice and practice to theories, and (c) provide guidelines for identifying and resolving clinical problems. The ultimate purpose is to use the most valid theories available as the foundation for assisting clients. The purpose of theory, on the other hand, is to (a) identify the characteristics of, and the relationships between, phenomena and (b) establish general principles that will expand our knowledge of the physical universe.

Application Sets of guidelines for practice are designed specifically to be applied. They provide direction for how to engage in problem identification and resolution with clients. Theories are not meant to be—nor can they be—directly used. They are descriptive only, exist separate from their use, and provide no suggestion for application.

Acceptance Sets of guidelines for practice are accepted by a profession to the extent to which they are considered adequate—that is, safe, effective, and efficient in problem identification and resolution and acceptable to clients. The latter refers to such factors as the amount of physical and/or mental distress associated with a client's participation in the process of problem identification and resolution stipulated in a set of guidelines. The adequacy of sets of guidelines for practice are specific to identified populations. Theories, on the other hand, are accepted or considered valid to the extent that they allow for accurate prediction about the phenomena they address.

Applied Type II Inquiry The four characteristics used to differentiate applied Type I inquiry from basic inquiry can also be employed to describe applied Type II inquiry (Allen, 1974; Broudy, Ennis, & Krimerman, 1973; Bunge, 1983;

Carroll, 1968; Downs, 1979; Feibleman 1983; Grove, 1989; Marx & Cronan-Hillix, 1987; Merton, 1982; Mosey, 1989; Scott & Shore, 1979; Vockell, 1983; Williams, 1974a).

The Fundamental Question

The fundamental question in applied Type II inquiry is: "What is the answer to this specific practical question?" Unlike basic inquiry, there is no intent to gain greater knowledge about the phenomena beyond the practical question being addressed.

The Goal

The immediate goal of applied Type II inquiry is to find the most accurate answer to the practical question being posed. In contrast, the goal of basic inquiry is to gain a broad and deep understanding of phenomena for the ultimate purpose of establishing general principles—that is, of articulating theory.

When applied Type II inquiry is used in conjunction with Type I inquiry, the questions posed are related to refining and assessing the adequacy of sets of guidelines for action. Thus, the ultimate goal is to determine to what extent sets of guidelines for action are adequate.

When applied Type II inquiry is addressed to practical questions other than those related to sets of guidelines for action, the goal is limited to finding the most accurate answer. Applied Type II inquiry is not concerned with how information is used per se because that would involve a decision-making process outside the boundaries of applied Type II inquiry. Decisions regarding the use of information are often influenced by a variety of factors in addition to the findings, such as financial or political considerations (Diesing, 1982; Rule, 1978; Scott & Shore, 1979).

Goals of inquiry imply motive or intent. One of the major differences between applied Type II inquiry and basic inquiry is the intent of the investigator. An individual engaged in applied Type II inquiry seeks to answer a practical question, limiting his of her study to that question. In contrast, an investigator engaged in basic inquiry seeks to broaden understanding of particular phenomena through developing, refining, or testing a theory. Because intent is a major factor in differentiating applied Type II inquiry from basic inquiry, an investigator must have the purpose of the task clearly delineated prior to initiating either form of inquiry. The purpose clearly influences all aspects of inquiry: what literature is reviewed, the way research questions are formed and posed, how hypotheses are stated, which research design is selected, and how findings are interpreted.

When the purpose of scientific inquiry is vague, the empirical data generated are likely to be isolated from any larger whole and be without context and, often, without meaning. It is rare that such findings contribute to answering a practical question or to formulating a theory. An investigator who does not know whether he or she is engaging in applied Type II inquiry or basic inquiry is like a person going into a kitchen to bake without knowing whether one's efforts are directed toward making a pie or a loaf of bread. Something may come out of the kitchen, but who knows what it will be?

The confusion between applied Type II inquiry and basic inquiry evident in some of the health professions exists regardless of whether a profession has a neopositivistic or disciplinal epistemological orientation. In research projects reported by different professions, it is often difficult to identify whether the project is applied Type II inquiry or basic inquiry. This may be due to several factors:

1. Lack of knowledge about the nature of the differences between applied Type II inquiry and basic inquiry.

2. The tendency to "do research" rather than engage in scientific inquiry. Participating in a research project is mistakenly equated with scientific inquiry. This confusion has been identified as a major deficit in the scientific work of both disciplines and professions (Rollin, 1988; Van Melsen, 1961; Williams, 1974b).

3. The belief that basic inquiry is "better" than applied inquiry. This results in labeling most scientific inquiry as basic when much of it is applied Type II inquiry.

4. The difficulty in stating the purpose of a research project beyond the project at hand.

This confusion creates fuzzy, rather than focused, research projects and scientific inquiry. The body of information generated by some professions tends to consist of isolated pieces of information without coherence or organization. There is no evidence of a larger context related either to sets of guidelines for practice being refined and assessed or to theories being developed and tested. No one synthesizes findings from a number of research projects. This is unfortunate because much of this information could be integrated and ultimately prove quite useful to a profession.

Occasionally, a particular research project is specifically designed to include both kinds of inquiry. However, such research projects are fairly rare, both because of their complexity and because of the difficulty involved in making them sufficiently focused to lead to the desired results. The area of gray between applied Type II inquiry and basic inquiry is far narrower than many people want to believe. Only by understanding the differences between applied Type II inquiry and basic inquiry can one combine these two kinds of scientific inquiry in a fruitful manner.

Process of Inquiry   As indicated in its definition, applied Type II inquiry involves use of the methods of science and research designs. Quantitative and qualitative research designs and their various subtypes—experimental and survey, ethnographic and case study, for example—are employed. The type of research design used depends on the question being addressed. When quantitative research designs are used, the process is similar in many ways to testing hypotheses as outlined in Chapter 8. Only the process is similar, however, not the intent or purpose of the study.

Product of Inquiry   The end product of applied Type II inquiry is empirical data—that is, postulates developed through the use of the methods and research designs of science. Given this definition, there is no difference between (a) the empirical data that are generated through basic inquiry in the process of developing, refining, and testing theories, and (b) the empirical data that are generated through applied Type II inquiry in the process of refining and assessing the adequacy of sets of guidelines for practice and in seeking answers to practical questions unrelated to sets of guidelines for action.

However, empirical data generated through applied Type II inquiry are rarely employed in developing theories or sets of guidelines for practice because they do not provide a viable foundation for sets of guidelines for practice nor information that enhances our fundamental knowledge of the physical universe. In general, the information is not found to be useful because:

1. The questions addressed are of a far more superficial nature than those addressed in basic inquiry.

2. The phenomena of concern are particular to the question addressed rather than representative of a larger category of phenomena.

3. It does not provide sufficient understanding for answering questions related to the "what" and "how" of phenomena.

Although the information generated by applied Type II inquiry is not typically used to develop theories or guidelines for action, this in no way negates the importance of applied Type II inquiry. Empirical data generated through applied Type II inquiry are included in the pool of "theoretical information," which is used as part of the theoretical foundation for sets of guidelines for practice and in the process of formulating theories.

In regards to theory development, empirical data generated through applied Type II inquiry are most often used indirectly, providing ideas that serve as the point of departure for theory development or as temporary support for an emerging theory. For instance, taking the United States census involves the use of applied Type II inquiry. The empirical data generated by each census become part of our pool of theoretical information. Scientists interested in developing a theory of human migration, for example, may use some of this empirical data as they engage in basic inquiry. Considerable additional phenomena would be included in such a theory and would need to be studied. The theory would then be tested postulate by postulate as outlined in Chapter 8.

Figure 7 provides a schematic representation of the relationship among the forms of scientific inquiry,

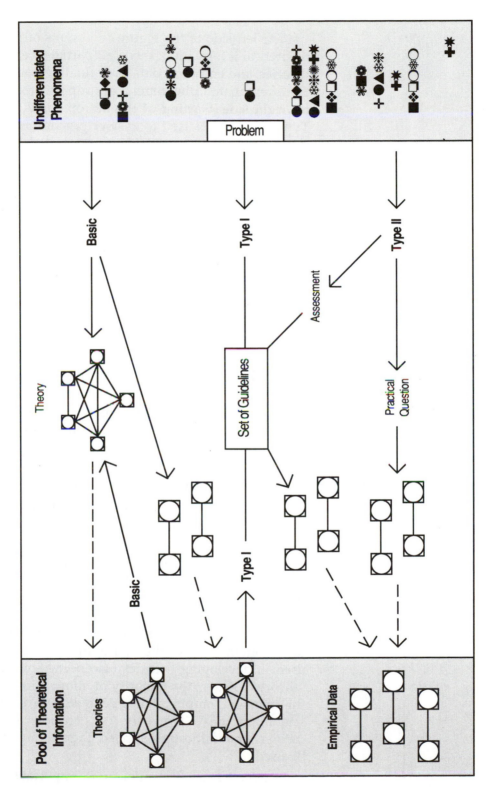

Figure 7: The relationship between basic, applied Type I, and applied Type II scientific inquiry; information generated by such inquiry; and use of that information.

the information generated by such inquiries, and the use of that information.

The left side of the Figure represents our pool of theoretical information: theories, partial or emerging theories, and empirical data (free-floating postulates). Undifferentiated phenomena are represented on the far right side. Starting at the bottom right, applied Type II inquiry is used to answer practical questions (solid line). The empirical data generated becomes part of the pool of theoretical information (broken line). Applied Type II inquiry is also used to refine and assess the adequacy of sets of guidelines for action (center of figure), leading to more empirical data added to the pool of theoretical information.

Applied Type I inquiry (left center of the figure) does not contribute to the pool of theoretical information. Rather, it draws upon the pool in order to develop sets of guidelines for practice. The information used most often is that generated through basic inquiry, not applied Type II inquiry. Sets of guidelines for practice are concerned with practical problems, hence the line from "problem" on the left side of the Figure. The line bracketing "Sets of Guidelines" represents the intimate connection between the problem, which forms the nucleus of sets of guidelines for practice, and theoretical information.

Basic inquiry may lead directly from undifferentiated phenomena to the development of theories, indicated on the upper right of Figure 7. These theories are added to the pool of theoretical information (broken line). Basic inquiry may also generate empirical data that cannot yet be integrated into the formal structure of theory (descending line from "Basic" on the right side). This information is also added to the pool of theoretical information.

Finally, in the process of basic inquiry, empirical data from the pool of theoretical information may be used in developing theories (ascending solid line to "theory"). Again, the majority of information used in this manner is empirical data generated through basic scientific inquiry. However, on occasion, empirical data generated through applied Type II inquiry may be used.

Applied Type II inquiry is an important part of

this endeavor we call science. It has and will continue to contribute to the conduct of human affairs. To confuse applied Type II inquiry with basic inquiry dilutes the significance of both and sharply impedes focused, goal-directed scientific inquiry.

Interactions between Applied Type I, Applied Type II, and Basic Scientific Inquiry

Various interactions between applied Type I, applied Type II, and basic scientific inquiry have been described above. However, controversy exists in the literature about the interactions between applied and basic inquiry. Some say there is no interaction because the modes of inquiry are in entirely different realms; others argue that they are on a continuum with one blending into the other. The interactions between applied Type I, applied Type II, and basic inquiry are more complex than either of these extreme points of view indicates.

Interactions among the modes of inquiry are described by diagramming and discussing seven typical scenarios.[1] There are other scenarios, and any large scientific project may involve various combinations of the scenarios described. For the sake of brevity, "problem" (as in clinical or technical problems) is used in this section when referring to applied Type I inquiry, and "question" when referring to applied Type II inquiry.

Scenario One

Raw, undifferentiated phenomena —> Basic inquiry —> Theory —>

(a) **Theory may or may not be valid.**

(b) **Theory may or may not be used as the basis for a set of guidelines for action at some later point.**

This scenario was described in Chapter 8. Raw, undifferentiated phenomena are subjected to basic

---

[1] The interactions to be described draw upon the work of Ausubel, 1953; Bouton, 1989; Branscomb, 1973; Brooks, 1988; Bunge, 1983; Feibleman, 1983; Fleming, Johnson, Marina, Spergel, and Townson, 1987; Foss and Rothenberg, 1987; Henderson, 1988; Kneller, 1978; Rosenberg and Birdzell, 1990; Scott and Shore, 1979; Vockell, 1983; Van Melsen, 1961; Wulff, Pedersen, and Rosenberg, 1986.

scientific inquiry, and a theory is developed, refined, and tested to determine its degree of validity. The theory is independent from its possible usefulness; it may or may not be suitable as the foundation for a set of guidelines for action. Whether a theory is or is not practically applied is in no way related to the theory's degree of validity.

Scenario Two

Problem —> Type I inquiry —> Set of guidelines for action —> Type II inquiry —> Findings —>

    (a) Set of guidelines is adequate; process ends.

    (b) Set of guidelines is inadequate —> continued Type II inquiry, or Type I inquiry is reinitiated.

In neither case has theoretical information been tested.

One or more theories and/or pieces of empirical data are used to develop a set of guidelines for action (applied Type I inquiry). The process of developing a set of guidelines begins either with a problem or with theoretical information. Whatever the point of departure, the remaining process is the same: the set of guidelines is refined and its adequacy assessed (applied Type II inquiry). When the set of guidelines is found to be adequate, further inquiry is not necessary—at least at this point. When found to be inadequate, the set of guidelines is further refined and assessed, or it is discarded. In the latter case, the process may begin all over again with applied Type I inquiry.

Regardless of whether a set of guidelines for action is found to be effective or ineffective, the theoretical information fundamental to it has *not* been tested in this process. This position is based on five premises:

Premise 1: Theoretical information may not be valid, yet the set of guidelines developed from that information may be effective. For example, theoretical information indicated that vapors arising from stagnant water were the cause of malaria. The effective set of guidelines developed to combat malaria was based in part on this information, but only later was it discovered that a parasitic protozoan transmitted through the bite of a mosquito causes malaria, not vapors from stagnant water.

From one perspective, the relationship between

theoretical information and a set of guidelines for action is a correlative relationship. In a correlation, one phenomenon is seen as varying in a particular manner relative to another phenomenon. Directional causality between them is neither implied nor assumed; there is always the possibility that covariance is due to a third factor. The same is true of theoretical information and a set of guidelines. The set of guidelines may be effective as the result of an unknown "third factor," not because the supporting theoretical information is valid.

Premise 2: Theoretical information fundamental to a set of guidelines for practice may be regarded as valid, yet the set of guidelines may be ineffective. For instance, if one uses a set of guidelines for practice based on operant conditioning to deal with disruptive behavior by adolescent spinal-cord-injured clients on a given rehabilitation unit and there is no change in their behavior, then it is apparent that the problem must be dealt with in another manner, perhaps one that focuses on the anxiety, anger, and frustration of these young people. Many factors may contribute to the ineffectiveness of this set of guidelines for practice—clients may have "seen through" the plan and were able to undermine it, or ethical constraints may have limited how rigorously the set of guidelines was implemented. The lack of effectiveness of this set of guidelines for this population in this rehabilitation unit says nothing about the validity of operant conditioning.

Premises 1 and 2 can be summarized as follows:

A. 1. Valid theoretical information may lead to an effective set of guidelines for action.

   2. Valid theoretical information may lead to an ineffective set of guidelines for action.

B. 1. Invalid theoretical information may lead to an effective set of guidelines for action.

   2. Invalid theoretical information may lead to an ineffective set of guidelines for action.

If these statements are accepted, it is a reasonable conclusion that testing the effectiveness of a theoretically based set of guidelines for action should not be construed as testing the validity of the theoretical information on which it is based.

Premise 3: If assessing the effectiveness of a set of guidelines for action was a test of the theoretical information fundamental to it, then any theoretical information could be identified as supporting an effective atheoretical set of guidelines and, thus, be considered valid. In other words, any proposed theory X, no matter how strange, could be offered as theoretical support for an atheoretical set of guidelines. As the set of guidelines has already been identified as effective, Theory X must be valid. Few scientists would accept this means of testing Theory X or any similar theoretical information. An example illustrating this can be found in the more than 200-year search for theoretical support for the effectiveness of aspirin and related drugs in reducing inflammation, swelling, and pain (Weissman, 1991). Edmund Stone documented the salutary effects of extracts of willow bark (later identified as salicylic acid) on febrile disorders in 1763. As theoretical support, he offered the "doctrine of signatures"—many natural maladies carry their cures along with them, or their remedies lie not far from their cause. Feverish illness and willow trees were both common in the area of England where Stone lived. This piece of empirical information was considered valid for a period of time. Subsequently, other theoretical explanations were offered and eventually rejected over the years. As recently as the early 1970s, it was proposed that salicylate blocked the local production of prostaglandin, minimizing inflammation. This was later found not to be the case. The latest postulate is that aspirin-like drugs are antiinflammatory because of their inhibitory effect on neutrophils, cells that are abundant in acute inflammation. Whether this postulate is valid is not yet known. However, its validity cannot be determined by assessing whether aspirin reduces inflammation.

Premise 4: Many sets of guidelines for action are derived from two or more theories and/or several pieces of empirical data. In assessing the effectiveness of such a set of guidelines, it is not possible to determine which aspects of the theoretical information have contributed to effectiveness. For example, a set of guidelines for practice concerned with supporting and facilitating mourning might be based on a theory regarding stages of mourning as well as some aspects of a theory of group dynamics. In assessing the effectiveness of this set of guidelines, it would be very difficult to know which theory was being tested. Testing the validity of either or both theories in this manner would produce highly contaminated research findings, negating sound interpretation.

Premise 5: Assessment of a set of guidelines for action usually takes place in a situation where there are a number of unknown or uncontrolled variables. It is difficult enough to assess a set of guidelines with any degree of confidence in such situations, but to also attempt to make knowledgeable interpretations about the validity of the theoretical information supporting the set of guidelines would be unwise. Theoretical information is best tested in a reasonably controlled situation through the use of basic inquiry.

The premises indicate that assessing the effectiveness of a set of guidelines for action should not be construed as testing the validity of its supporting theoretical information.

Scenario Three

Problem —> Type I inquiry —> No theoretical information —> Basic inquiry —>

(a) **Formulate suitable theoretical information —> Type I inquiry —> proceed as in Scenario Two.**

(b) **Suitable theoretical information cannot be formulated —> seek other solutions.**

In this scenario, applied Type I inquiry is used to investigate a given problem. However, no theories or empirical data are found to support development of a set of guidelines for action. Basic inquiry is then brought to bear on the phenomena thought to underlie the problem. If suitable theoretical information is formulated, a set of guidelines for action is developed following Scenario Two.

In the situation described in the first part of this scenario, basic and applied scientific inquiry may be so closely interrelated in time and place that the line between the two processes seems to blur. This happens especially when there is a pressing need to fabricate a particular technological product, such as the polio vaccine. However, basic scientific inquiry, engaged in for the express purpose of gaining knowledge that can ultimately be used as the foundation for a set of guidelines for action, is still basic inquiry. It remains concerned with identifying basic principles about the nature of the physical universe. The knowledge gained through this kind of "focused" basic inquiry cannot be directly used; applied Type I inquiry must be employed before the theoretical information can serve as the basis for a set of guidelines for action. Moreover, applied inquiry of either type—no matter how elegant or complex—never becomes basic inquiry. It is concerned only with resolution of practical problems or finding answers to practical questions.

When suitable theoretical information cannot be formulated to support development of a set of guidelines for action, other ways of dealing with the problem must be found. One common solution is to attempt to formulate an atheoretical set of guidelines for action through practical inquiry. Another solution, used particularly in the health professions, is to work around the target problem by formulating theoretically based sets of guidelines for practice directed toward problems that are associated with the target problem. This is discussed in more detail in Chapter 10.

Scenario Four

An atheoretical set of guidelines —> Type I inquiry —>

    (a) Theoretical information identified —> set of guidelines becomes theoretically based.

    (b) No theoretical information —> basic inquiry.

Atheoretical sets of guidelines for action are formulated through practical inquiry without reference to theoretical information. This is exemplified in the set of technological guidelines used to make high temperature superconductors. As of this writing, there is no theory to support these guidelines. Similarly, the set of guidelines for practice developed by the Bobaths (1979) dealing with abnormal patterns of movement as a consequence of central nervous system deficit (used in physical and occupational therapy) has little, if any, valid theoretical support. Sets of technological guidelines for fabricating therapeutic drugs are also sometimes formulated through practical inquiry.

Other atheoretical sets of guidelines for action may have been originally formulated through applied Type

I and Type II inquiry and found to be effective. However, after their successful formulation, the supporting theoretical information is determined to be invalid. The sets of guidelines become atheoretical by default, yet they continue to be used because they are effective. Electroshock therapy (EST), used to treat severe depression, is a prominent example. The original empirical data supporting EST indicated that individuals who had seizures rarely, if ever, had psychotic disorders. These data have long since been recognized as invalid.

Applied Type I inquiry is used to identify the theoretical foundation of an effective atheoretical set of guidelines for action for two reasons. One is simple curiosity, the desire to know more about the phenomena and why the set of guidelines is effective. Second, understanding the theoretical base of an atheoretical set of guidelines allows the set of guidelines to be furthered refined and made safer, more effective, efficient, and acceptable to clients. When supporting theoretical information is identified, the set of guidelines for action becomes theoretically based.

At times, applied Type I inquiry of an atheoretical set of guidelines for action is not fruitful because no theoretical information can be found to support the set of guidelines. As in Scenario Three, basic inquiry addressing the underlying phenomena involved is required. Such study is currently taking place, for example, with regard to high temperature superconductors and electroshock therapy.

Scenario Five

Question —> Type II inquiry —> Findings —>

(a) **Answers question; process ends.**

(b) **Raises many questions —> for those who are interested, process shifts to basic inquiry —> theoretical information.**

In applied Type II inquiry, a practical question is addressed with the intent of finding an answer—or at least a partial answer. Additional applied Type II inquiry may take place to arrive at a more complete or definitive answer. This process ends when the question has been answered to the satisfaction of those posing the question or to the extent that resources permit. The focus is always on the practical question with no concern about theory development.

Sometimes the course of applied Type II inquiry leads to speculation of a broader nature. If investigators redirect their attention to the study of phenomena underlying the original question for the purpose of theory development, the goal of their inquiry has changed and they are engaging in basic scientific inquiry. For example, if a school district has funds to buy new playground equipment, the needs and interests of special students must be considered before deciding what to purchase. One question is: "What playground equipment is now used most frequently by orthopedically impaired children in the school district?" This question is addressed through applied Type II inquiry, but, in the course of the study, the investigator may begin to think about the nature of gross motor development, exploratory play, and the use of toys and equipment that are immediately available in the environment. If this speculation leads to a series of projects designed to study these phenomena and their relationships to each other, the investigator has shifted to basic scientific inquiry.

Applied Type II inquiry is not concerned with promoting interest in theory development. Any movement into basic inquiry is a minor offshoot that occasionally happens. In theory development, individuals interested in extensive, in-depth study of a phenomenon start with basic scientific inquiry.

Scenario Six

Assessment tool (problem) —> Type I inquiry —> Tentative tool —> Type II inquiry —>

(a) Tool with good reliability and validity.

(b) Tool with minimal reliability and validity.

"Assessment tool" refers to a broad category of procedures or methods employed for gaining information. Examples include personality and intelligence tests, screening tools used in the health professions, predictive tools used for some kinds of placement, and tools specially designed for a research project involving basic or applied Type II inquiry. Specifically excluded from this list are tools used for problem identification that are part of a set of guidelines for practice. Development of these kinds of tools is discussed in Chapter 10, as are the issues of reliability and validity of assessment tools.

Applied Scientific Inquiry in the Health Professions

Some assessment tools are theoretically based, developed initially through the use of applied Type I inquiry. Theoretical information is used to identify the nature and scope of the phenomena to be assessed by the tool. For example, in developing an intelligence test, an investigator goes to the theoretical literature to identify what is meant by "intelligence," what is typically included in the definition of intelligence on an abstract level, and, perhaps, what behaviors are associated with various degrees and/or kinds of intelligence. With suitable theoretical information in hand, the investigator begins to design a tool for assessment. Subsequent or simultaneous applied Type II inquiry helps refine and establish the reliability and validity of the tool. This brief overview of developing adequate assessment tools simplifies a difficult and lengthy process.

Scenario Seven

[Problem —> Type I inquiry —> Technological guidelines] —> Technological product —> Type II inquiry —>

(a) Enhancement of basic inquiry —> theory.

(b) Enhancement of Type II inquiry —> more refined, complete answers.

This final scenario involves the use of technological products to facilitate the work of basic and applied scientific inquiry. The first part of the diagram is bracketed to indicate that a technological product may be derived from applied Type I inquiry, making the technological guidelines for creating the product theoretically based. While this is often the case, atheoretical sets of guidelines developed through practical inquiry may also be used to make a technological product.

Technological products employed in basic inquiry typically are tools that enhance observation, manipulation, and measurement of phenomena or the treatment of data—telescopes and thermometers, for instance. Some technological products are developed specifically for use in basic inquiry, such as supercolliders. Others are originally developed to facilitate basic inquiry but have found broader application, such as lasers. Technological products fabricated from theoretically based sets of guidelines have had a significant effect on the advancement of basic science.

Without these products, our knowledge of the physical universe would be far less than it is today.

Technological products have also contributed to the advancement of applied Type II inquiry. The use of computers to process data, for instance, makes it easier to examine more data with greater efficiency.

In summary, there are many and varied relationships between basic, applied Type I, and applied Type II scientific inquiries. Each contributes to and enhances the others, yet each is separate and distinct.

10. *Formulating Sets of Guidelines for Practice*

This chapter is concerned with formulating—developing, refining, and assessing the adequacy of—sets of guidelines for practice (Ausubel, 1953; Carroll, 1968; Feibleman, 1983; Horgan, 1988; Kneller, 1978; Marx & Cronan-Hillix, 1987; Mosey, 1986; Vockell, 1983; Wulff, Pedersen, & Rosenberg, 1986). It provides some fundamental principles of formulation, aspects of theoretical information to consider, and steps to take. Due to the differences among various health professions' sets of guidelines, the discussion of principles and steps will be necessarily general. The last section, "Some Observations...," offers suggestions of what to do when no apparent theoretical information exists to support the formulation of a set of guidelines for practice. This is followed by discussion of common difficulties associated with sets of guidelines for practice.

Overview of the Process

The process of formulating a set of guidelines for practice is not linear but entails moving back and forth among various phases and steps within phases and between applied Type I and Type II inquiry. A set of guidelines is formed, refined, and assessed throughout the process. Figure 8 illustrates this circular process; the arrows, starting at clinical observation, indicate the ultimate flow of events.

As the diagram illustrates, the entire process is grounded in clinical observation. Astute observation

Figure 8. Schematic representation of development, refinement, and assessment of the adequacy of sets of guidelines for practice using applied Type I and Type II scientific inquiry.

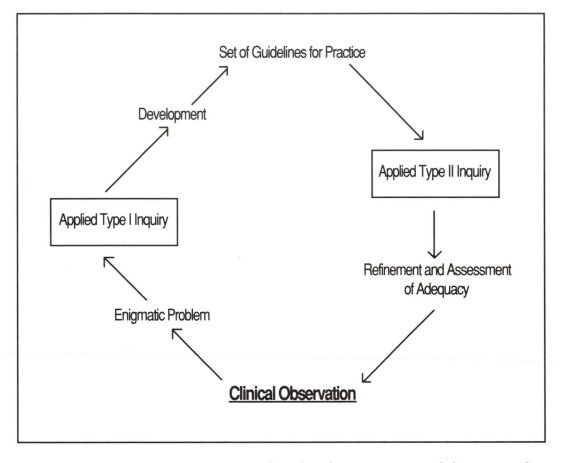

is essential to the ultimate success of the process because a set of guidelines for practice is likely to match the problem it is designed to identify and resolve only when its entire formulation takes place in the context of clinical observation. It is through clinical observation that practitioners become aware of problems for which sets of guidelines for practice need to be developed. Refining and assessing the adequacy of sets of guidelines for practice require careful observation of their use in the clinical setting. Without sensitive, perceptive observation, formulating sets of guidelines becomes an intellectual exercise divorced from clinical practice.

The point of departure for formulating a set of guidelines for practice is typically an *enigmatic problem*—a clinical condition or situation of a client that is

Applied Scientific Inquiry in the Health Professions

puzzling or inexplicable to the profession and cannot be adequately addressed by existing sets of guidelines. An enigmatic problem may be a condition or situation that (a) has not previously existed, (b) is new to the profession (c) has not been recognized before, (d) is resistive to adequate resolution, or (e) is now dealt with through use of an atheoretical set of guidelines.

Occasionally, theoretical information is the starting point for the process of formulating sets of guidelines for practice. A practitioner becomes aware of new or revised theories or empirical data that appear to have potential for use in a set of guidelines. Study of the theoretical information may lead to recognition of an enigmatic problem or to reconsideration of a generally accepted set of guidelines. The new theoretical information changes one's perspective, allowing for the possibility of different, more adequate approaches.

Whether one begins with an enigmatic problem or theoretical information, the remaining parts of the process are quite similar. The only advantage of beginning with theoretical information is that the step, "identification of useful theories and empirical data," has already been initiated.

The first phase of formulating a set of guidelines for practice is development, which involves the use of applied Type I inquiry. The nature of the problem is elucidated, the elements of the problem clarified, and the possible means of problem resolution outlined. Some preliminary refinement of the tentative set of guidelines for practice takes place relative to consideration of internal consistency and completeness of content.

The second phase involves the use of applied Type II inquiry and is concerned with refining and assessing the adequacy of sets of guidelines for practice (see the right side of Figure 8). Attention is given to such issues as reliability and validity of problem identification, specificity of the guidelines for problem resolution, safety, and effectiveness.

The two phases—and all of the steps within these phases—are described in the remaining sections of the chapter. Because some of the explanations are a bit lengthy, the reader may find that periodically referring back to Figure 8 is helpful.

Developing a Set of Guidelines

As outlined in Chapter 9—and now specific to sets of guidelines for practice—applied Type I inquiry involves five steps:

1. Analysis of an enigmatic problem.
2. Identification of suitable theories/empirical data.
3. Selection and synthesis of germane postulates to form a theoretical foundation.
4. Deduction, from the theoretical foundation, of:
   a. Guidelines for problem identification.
   b. Guidelines for problem resolution.
5. Consideration of internal consistency and completeness of content.

Analysis of an Enigmatic Problem

In this description, the development of sets of guidelines for practice begins with an enigmatic problem. Analysis of an enigmatic problem involves dissecting the problem in such a way that one begins to understand some of its characteristics. Often, however, no analytic framework exists to provide guidance or even clues. One must feel one's way through the problem. The goal is to gain sufficient preliminary understanding so that one has some idea of where to start looking for theoretical information. Clinical observation is of primary importance: talking with clients who manifest the problem, observing their behavior, surveying any available laboratory findings, and reading case histories. Consultation with professional colleagues and other team members is also helpful.

Some questions to guide analysis include:

1. What are the characteristics of the enigmatic problem?
2. What systems are involved: biological, psychological, cognitive, aspects of daily functioning?
3. What primary and secondary diagnostic categories and other problems are associated with the enigmatic problem?
4. Are there commonalities in the demographic data or life situation of clients with the problem?
5. What are possible causal factors?

The ideas that are generated provide at least initial direction for a search of the literature. Many more questions will be raised as analysis continues.

Identification of Suitable Theories/ Empirical Data

For this step, identification of theories/empirical data, understanding theory is imperative. Although one may find considerable theoretical information, it is the ability to determine the suitability of the information that is important. Suitability of theoretical information refers to (a) relevance to the enigmatic problem being considered, (b) relative simplicity, (c) structural adequacy, (d) degree of validity, and (e) compatibility with the profession's fundamental body of knowledge.

Relevant theoretical knowledge comes in two forms. Static theoretical information elucidates the problem, "the nature of the thing," its component parts, and the associated behaviors and physical signs. Dynamic information is also sought—that is, factors that may impinge upon, lead to, alter in some way, or ameliorate the problem. Causal factors sometimes contribute to greater understanding of the problem, but they may not be useful in developing sets of guidelines for practice.

Theoretical explanations should be straightforward and have a relative simplicity rather than being complex and elaborate. Simple theoretical explanations are likely to be more useful in developing sets of guidelines for practice. Occam's razor should be wielded skillfully in the process of selecting suitable theories/empirical data.

Structurally adequate theoretical information is more likely to be useful than information with serious structural deficits. Completeness and specificity of definitions are probably the most important structural components to consider. Theoretical information can rarely serve as the foundation for a set of guidelines for practice when concepts are not well-defined. Simple concepts or constructs that can be easily defined operationally enhance the usefulness of theoretical information. Postulates should clearly and explicitly identify the relationship between concepts.

The degree of empirical validity of promising theoretical information needs to be determined; this may be done in comparison with other theoretical information about the same phenomena, if any is available. Theoretical information that has only considerable face validity may be suitable for developing sets of guidelines for practice but should be used with caution.

Finally, attention is given to the compatibility of potentially suitable theories and empirical data with the profession's fundamental body of knowledge—especially regarding the profession's philosophical assumptions, code of ethics, and legitimate tools. As the theoretical information is considered, the investigator begins to form a tentative set of guidelines for practice, thereby getting a sense of what the set of guidelines might look like if information from one theoretical system is used over information from another. During this process, questions such as these are asked relative to the profession's philosophical assumptions and code of ethics:

1. Would this tentative set of guidelines be compatible with the profession's goals and view of the individual?

2. Would the process of problem identification and resolution be within the bounds of the profession's ethical standards?

For example, one may consider using postulates drawn from two different learning theories: classical conditioning and operant conditioning. Some professions may feel that a set of guidelines for practice based on classical conditioning would be demeaning to individuals and, therefore, suspect relative to the profession's code of ethics. In this case, postulates from operant conditioning may be selected for use in the developing set of guidelines for practice.

A profession's legitimate tools limit to some extent what theories and empirical data are suitable for use in a set of guidelines for practice. In considering theoretical information, an investigator should ask the question: "Would a set of guidelines based on this theoretical information be compatible with, and/or provide direction for, use of the profession's legitimate tools?" Theoretical information emphasizing the biochemical aspects of a problem would not be compatible with the legitimate tools of social work, for example, but would be compatible with those of medicine. The reverse would be true for theoretical information suggesting that living conditions were a factor affecting the problem.

At some point during the analysis of the enigmatic problem and the study of theories/empirical data, the investigator decides whether the enigmatic problem will be treated as a single entity or as made up of two or more components. For example, "stress reduction," a single entity, may be broken down into such sub-problems as "recognition of the experience of stress," "identification of stressful situations," and "consideration of possible stress reduction activities." This determination greatly affects how the problem will be approached. The general rule is that when part of the problem may be dealt with separate from other parts, the problem should be treated as having multiple components. Developing sets of guidelines for practice for a problem treated as a single entity is described here. Sets of guidelines for practice with multiple components are discussed in Chapter 11.

The search for suitable theories and empirical data is detective work—one seeks clues and pieces together bits of information. It is a tedious, often time-consuming task, but one that may prove very rewarding.

Selection and Synthesis of Germane Postulates to Form a Theoretical Foundation

This step in the process of developing sets of guidelines for practice is concerned with selecting postulates, not isolated concepts disconnected from the structure of a postulate. Isolated concepts are usually not used because a category of phenomena has little meaning when it is unrelated to other categories of phenomena and is outside of some larger context.

A theory is rarely used in its entirety in a set of guidelines for practice. Rather, only those postulates germane to the enigmatic problem are selected from theories. Ideally, the rule of parsimony is rigorously followed; only essential postulates are chosen. Commonly, postulates are selected from two or more theories and various pieces of empirical data. Prior to combining such disparate information, one must consider the compatibility of the basic assumptions underlying the various pieces of theoretical information. For example, psychoanalytically oriented theories and learning theories with a behavioral focus are based on different assumptions regarding human behavior. In the former, intrapsychic content is considered to be the major factor influencing behavior, while in the latter behavior is considered to be influenced primarily by interaction with the external environment. Combining pieces of theoretical information with incompatible basic assumptions is difficult and usually unnecessary.

A second possible impediment to successfully combining disparate theoretical information is the possibility of concept definition-label inconsistency. For example, if an investigator finds one concept with two different labels, he or she must select one for use in the set of guidelines for practice. If two different concepts have the same label, and both concepts are to be used, the label of one must be changed. Or, two concepts with the same label may be defined slightly differently in two pieces of theoretical information. The investigator must decide whether the difference is substantive or superficial. In any event, the basic substance or essence of a concept definition should never be changed, and relabeling concepts should be avoided, if at all possible.

Third, compatibility of focus along the biological-behavioral continuum must be assessed. Pieces of theoretical information with different foci should be combined with care. The tendency, for example, to equate perceptual/cognitive behavior with neurological structures and processes is somewhat risky given our present state of knowledge. Similarly, it is difficult to combine information from neurodevelopmental and biomechanical theories into one set of guidelines for practice.

The final requirement when synthesizing theoretical information is to conserve the contextual integrity of selected postulates. Using postulates out of context—out of the matrix that surrounds and influences their meaning—is not acceptable. Doing so changes the meaning of the postulate and its component concepts. While taking postulates out of context tends to be more of a problem with behavioral information than with biological information, it is a factor to consider regardless of theoretical focus.

After due consideration of the above factors, the selected postulates are synthesized in some manner (see Chapter 11 for further elaboration), and they become the theoretical foundation of the set of guidelines for practice. The form of the theoretical foundation is dependent on the needs of a profession, but, whatever the form, the relationship between postulates must be stated and the theoretical foundation integrated into a whole. As always, all concepts must be adequately defined.

By this point, the enigmatic problem has usually been given a name, making it less mysterious—although little may be known about it yet.

Deduction of Guidelines for Problem Identification and Resolution

Developing *guidelines for problem identification* involves the enumeration of problem indicators—that is, the behaviors (actions and verbal reports) and physical signs used to determine the presence of a problem. These are the signs and symptoms of diagnostic categories and the behaviors and physical signs indicative of function and dysfunction in frames of reference. Problem indicators are deduced from the theoretical foundation as well as from observation of the enigmatic problem.

Well-enumerated problem indicators have three major characteristics:

1. They are stated in such a way that the presence or absence of the problem can be differentiated from other related problems. Indicators that do not differentiate are superfluous, thus ignoring the rule of parsimony.

2. Indicators are stated so that it is clear what information is needed and how that information can be obtained. In other words, it should be fairly evident how one goes about the process of problem assessment with the client.

3. Problem indicators should be as specific and as directly observable as possible.

Guidelines for problem resolution are deduced from the theoretical base and consist of precepts stating the nature, quality, quantity, and sequence of interactions between client, practitioner, and the environment. Environment is used broadly to include (a) people other than the client and practitioner, as in the use of group interactions; (b) manmade and natural entities, such as music and food; and (c) specific technological products, such as splints and medication. Guidelines are stated as clearly as possible so that they can be followed by informed practitioners.

Care must be taken that the guidelines for resolution are addressed to the problem and not to problem indicators. Otherwise, the problem needs to be reassessed and the guidelines reconceptualized.

Consideration of Internal Consistency and Completeness of Content

The last step in developing a set of guidelines for practice is the consideration of internal consistency and completeness of content. *Internal consistency* refers to the congruence between the theoretical foundation and the other parts of the set of guidelines for practice. When information within the theoretical foundation is not used as the basis for guidelines for problem identification or resolution—indicating a lack of attention to the rule of parsimony—the unnecessary information should be deleted. On the other hand, occasionally information extraneous to the theoretical foundation is used as the basis for the guidelines.

Use of information not included in the theoretical foundation is to be avoided. When guidelines for problem identification and resolution are not derived solely from the theoretical foundation, the entire set of guidelines for practice needs to be reviewed.

Completeness of content refers to whether a set of guidelines for practice includes all the required information. Two question are relevant:

1. Is the set of guidelines for practice able to be used without recourse to extraneous information?

2. Does the set of guidelines for practice have sufficient information stated in such a manner that short- and long-term effects of application can be assessed?

The need for completeness of content will become apparent in discussion of refining and assessing the adequacy of sets of guidelines for practice; however, content should be as complete as possible prior to moving on to applied Type II inquiry.

Refining and Assessing the Adequacy of Sets of Guidelines for Practice

Once a tentative set of guidelines for practice is developed, the process begins to involve use of applied Type II inquiry. But because the process is not linear, one may need to return to one or more of the steps involved in applied Type I inquiry. Refining and assessing the adequacy of sets of guidelines for practice are typically conjoint processes—refinement being part of assessment, assessment leading to further refinement, further refinement necessitating additional assessment. Therefore, only occasionally in this discussion is any attempt made to separate these two activities.

There are many excellent textbooks concerned with designing reliable and valid evaluation procedures and conducting evaluative research. Their discussions of clinical evaluation are often couched strictly in terms of evaluation, although refinement is frequently the goal. These textbooks describe appropriate research designs and discuss methodological and ethical issues inherent in this kind of applied Type II inquiry. Readers are advised to consult such texts. The discussion here places this readily available information into the context of refining and assessing the adequacy of sets of guidelines for practice.

Refining and assessing the adequacy of guidelines for problem identification will be described first, followed by a consideration of guidelines for problem resolution. Although the process is often sequential as described here, it does not have to be.

Guidelines for Problem Identification

The purpose of refining and assessing the adequacy of guidelines for problem identification is to design reliable and valid procedures for evaluation.

In order for them to be useful in evaluation with a client, guidelines for problem identification must be reliable and valid. Evaluation procedures can be viewed as being on a continuum that ranges from using only problem indicators as outlined in a set of guidelines for practice (unstandardized) to developing standardized tests for inclusion in a set of guidelines for practice. *Standardized tests* are evaluation procedures characterized by control for administrator bias, specified conditions for administration and scoring, normative data, and a high degree of reliability and validity (Cronbach, 1985). Where the evaluative procedures for a given set of guidelines for practice are placed on this unstandardized-to-standardized continuum depends on:

1. How accurately and reliably an area of human function can be measured given the extent of inherent differences among individuals and

their particular situations.

2. How accurately and reliably an area of human function needs to be measured.

3. The resources (time, money, etc.) available for designing a standardized evaluation procedure.

Some practitioners believe that standardized tests are the best type of evaluation procedure. Although standardized tests are very useful in many areas, they should not be idealized. All areas of human function cannot be reduced to metric or quasi-metric proportion, and some people would say they should not be. When developing evaluation procedures, it is best to think in terms of what is possible, necessary, efficient, and acceptable to the client. That said, the following discussion is not concerned with the placement of an evaluation procedure on the unstandardized-to-standardized continuum.

The majority of evaluation procedures are based on two interrelated factors: (a) sampling of behavior and physical signs and (b) situational stimuli. Sampling is used because the entirety of behaviors and physical signs cannot be observed. For instance, one has time to observe a client's gait as he or she walks down the hall but not to watch the client walking in various places and situations throughout the day. Similarly, a test for cholesterol level involves the use of only a small amount of blood. Sampling determines the presence or absence of a problem—admittedly at some risk. Situational stimuli are what allow for the observation of the behavior and physical signs deemed necessary for problem identification. Requesting the client to walk down the hall is likely to be sufficient situational stimuli for an observation of gait. In determining cholesterol level, the initial stimulus is the prick of a needle, but more important are the stimuli used to arrive at an accurate reading of the cholesterol level.

Problem indicators, when properly stated in a set of guidelines for practice, provide a description of the behaviors and physical signs to be sampled and of the requisite situational stimuli. The latter are sometimes more implied than specifically stated. From these indicators, more formal or standardized evaluation procedures are designed, if necessary.

Evaluation procedures are only useful when they have a satisfactory degree of reliability and validity. Reliability means that an evaluation procedure leads to consistent findings. Although there are many types of reliability, the two usually considered of primary importance are "test-retest" and "interrater." Test-retest reliability refers to the extent to which similar results are obtained when an evaluation procedure is repeated. Interrater reliability refers to the degree of agreement between practitioners regarding the type of data gathered and the interpretation of that data.

When used in the context of evaluation procedures, validity means that the procedure measures what it reports to measure. Content validity, the most important form of validity, is the degree to which behavior and physical signs used in the procedure are representative of the area being assessed. It is established through a careful analysis of the area of human function to be assessed and of the design of the evaluation situation in order to determine the degree to which the procedure provides an adequate sample of the area being assessed. Establishing content validity is quite similar to identifying problem indicators, but it happens later in the process of developing a tentative set of guidelines for practice. Content validity is probably best assessed by individuals not originally involved in developing a set of guidelines. Other types of validity may also need to be established depending on the nature of the problem and type of evaluation procedure developed. Textbooks concerned with this issue should be consulted.

Evaluation procedures designed for a particular set of guidelines for practice are specific to that set of guidelines. Taking an evaluation procedure from one set of guidelines and using it for another is indefensible from a scholarly perspective, and, more practically, the "borrowed" procedure is not likely to be very useful.

There is a tendency in some health professions to develop evaluation tools that are unrelated to any set of guidelines for practice. Such tools, unless designed and used for the purpose of screening, are of little worth. Identifying problems and/or components of problems without even a tentative formulation of guidelines for problem resolution is a fruitless activity. Moreover, the way a problem is conceptualized is interrelated with its resolution. One would have great difficulty, for example, resolving a problem conceptualized in psychoanalytical terms through the use of behavioral modification techniques. Evaluation procedures, except those concerned with screening, should be developed and used only within the context of a set of guidelines for practice.

Guidelines for Problem Resolution

Some of the following factors involved in refining and assessing the adequacy of guidelines for problem resolution also pertain to guidelines for problem identification as well as to sets of guidelines for practice in general.

The first task is to determine whether the guidelines are stated clearly enough to be followed consistently by informed practitioners—that is, do the guidelines have interpractitioner reliability? This is established in much the same way as interrater reliability. The investigator explores the extent to which practitioners design and engage in similar intervention regimens with clients using only the particular guidelines in question. Until some degree of interpractitioner reliability is established, further assessment of guidelines for problem resolution would not be warranted.

Refining and assessing the adequacy of guidelines for problem resolution can be viewed as having four dimensions:

1. Specificity—when, how often, what amount, how long.

2. Efficacy—safety, effectiveness, efficiency, and acceptability to clients.

3. Context of use—alone, in combination with other sets of guidelines, and/or as one step in a sequence involving use of several sets of guidelines for practice.

4. In relationship to different populations.

These four dimensions are interrelated, as are all of their components.

Applied Scientific Inquiry in the Health Professions

Before discussing these dimensions, however, the place of probability in describing the adequacy of sets of guidelines for practice should be noted (Wulff, Pedersen, & Rosenberg, 1986). Probability is the relative possibility of an event occurring as expressed by the ratio of the number of actual occurrences of the event to the total number of possible occurrences. There are few absolutes in clinical practice. Individuals vary so widely and react to treatment so differently that little can be done in clinical practice with unqualified certainty. Therefore, in describing the adequacy of a set of guidelines for practice, such factors as length of treatment, safety, and acceptability to clients are able to be expressed only in terms of probability. Thus, we say that therapeutic drug X is effective for 98% of a given population. Whether this drug would be effective for a particular individual within this population is unknown. Regardless of the degree of probable adequacy under the four dimensions outlined, selection and use of a particular set of guidelines for practice are always matters of judgment on the part of the practitioner and the client.

Specificity
As has been mentioned, guidelines for problem resolution describe the nature, quality, quantity, and sequence of interactions. In assessing guidelines, these aspects of intervention are studied in more detail. While the questions used in assessments will vary, some common ones are:

1. When in the course of intervention should the guidelines for problem resolution be used? Immediately? During rehabilitation?

2. How often should the client be involved in the regimen outlined in the guidelines for problem resolution? Three times a day? Twice a week?

3. What amount or level of a therapeutic tool should be used? The dosage of a therapeutic drug prescribed? Heat applied? Calories recommended?

4. How long should the client engage in the regimen for maximal positive effect? Until it can be determined no positive effect is likely?

Efficacy
Efficacy, which includes safety, effectiveness, efficiency, and acceptability to clients, is the second di-

mension in refining and assessing guidelines for problem resolution.

Safety is of paramount importance. If application of guidelines for problem resolution is able to do good, so too may the guidelines do harm; if they are so innocuous that harm is highly unlikely, little good is likely either. In their concern for demonstrating effectiveness, health professionals sometimes do not give sufficient attention to the safety of their sets of guidelines for practice. Adequate safety consideration means assessing the possibility for harm or injury as well as the nature and degree of severity of any nontherapeutic effects. Contraindications should be identified. Refinements may make the guidelines for problem resolution safer for clients.

The *effectiveness* of guidelines for problem resolution is often considered from the perspective of time. Long-term effectiveness is usually seen as preferable, although short-term effectiveness may be all that is desired in some cases. Usually both short- and long-term effectiveness are assessed. The effectiveness of guidelines is compared (a) to other sets of guidelines concerned with the same problem, if any exist, and (b) to doing nothing. On the whole, practitioners want to do something. When doing nothing is found to be the most effective course of action, practitioners may be troubled.

Efficiency is concerned with the amount of time and energy expended by the client and practitioner. Sets of guidelines for practice are formulated to be as efficient as possible, and refinement may lead to greater efficiency. Efficiency is considered relative to other sets of guidelines for practice dealing with the same problem and to taking no action. Efficiency is often related solely to economic factors; however, it is more than that. The amount of effort the client is going to have to spend on problem resolution cannot be measured in economic terms alone.

Acceptability to clients is important to both guidelines for problem identification and guidelines for resolution. What amount of physical and/or mental distress is associated with a client's participation in the process as stipulated in the set of guidelines for practice? Congruence with the client's personal and cultural values is also of importance here. While these areas cannot be adequately measured in quantitative terms, they need to be honestly stated and assessed in some manner. Refining sets of guidelines for practice is directed towards increasing acceptability to clients whenever possible.

Context of Use

Sets of guidelines for practice are refined and assessed in terms of their use alone, their use in combination with other sets of guidelines, and their use in a sequence of different sets of guidelines for practice used over time. For example, set A, concerned with physical rehabilitation, may be fairly effective when used alone, but it may be more effective when used in combination with set B, which is directed towards minimizing frustration and anxiety. Moreover, set A may be more efficient when it is employed subsequent to the use of set C, concerned with minimizing pain. Because many clients have multiple problems, several sets of guidelines are often used at the same time. When assessing sets of guidelines for practice, it is important to determine how each set of guidelines can be employed to its best advantage in the context of many others.

Different Populations

Finally, sets of guidelines for practice are assessed in terms of different client populations. To a great extent, which population categories are selected for consideration depends upon the problem area addressed and the nature of the set of guidelines for practice. Various age groups are almost always considered. Other categories investigated may include gender, primary and secondary diagnosis, general state of physical or mental health, pregnancy or the possibility thereof, and motivation, to name a few. Refinement and assessment with regard to different populations are always conducted relative to the other three dimensions—specificity, efficacy, context of use—and their components. For example, the safety and effectiveness of a set of guidelines for practice need to be determined relative to different age groups, because what is safe and effective for one age group may not be for another.

In conclusion, refining and assessing the adequacy of a set of guidelines for practice are lengthy and, at times, tedious processes, but they must be done. One may develop an elegant set of guidelines that looks magnificent on paper, but until it is adequately assessed it remains just that—magnificent on paper. On the other hand, it is a poor use of time and resources to go through the process of refining and assessing a set of guidelines for practice that is based on questionably valid theoretical information, is incomplete, or is poorly stated. Skilled use of both applied Type I and II inquiry is necessary in formulating adequate sets of guidelines for practice.

Some Observations on Sets of Guidelines for Practice
When There Are No Theories or Empirical Data

Broaden the search.

On occasion, a practitioner is unable to find suitable, sufficiently valid theories or empirical data that will provide a theoretical foundation for a set of guidelines for practice. This may occur when attempting to formulate a set of guidelines for an enigmatic problem or when seeking theoretical support for an atheoretical set of guidelines. A number of actions can be taken when this happens:

It may be that one has not investigated enough or in the right places. A return to the literature may be in order: rereading what has already been read, seeking out less obvious sources, investigating literature that seems peripheral to the problem, and so forth. Talking with members of one's own profession, or of other related professions and appropriate disciplines may lead to clarification of the problem and identification of new sources for exploration.

Reexamine the enigmatic problem.

Something may have been missed in the original analysis. The problem may need to be looked at from another perspective or formulated in a different manner before returning to the literature. Many investigators do not take enough time to analyze an enigmatic problem because they rush to find a means of resolution before the problem has been adequately studied and understood.

Select less than suitable theories and empirical data as the foundations for a set of guidelines.

In other words, theoretical information that is not as valid, complete, specific, or as directly related to the enigmatic problem as one would like may be used as the basis for a set of guidelines for practice. A practitioner may have to make some questionable assumptions when using such information—for example, applying findings from animal studies to humans—or may need to engage in inductive reasoning that goes

Applied Scientific Inquiry in the Health Professions

beyond the usually accepted limits. When inadequate theories and empirical data are used as the basis for a set of guidelines, it must be acknowledged. This not only warns the user but also marks the set of guidelines for practice as one in need of further applied Type I inquiry.

Develop suitable theoretical information.

Occasionally, this is done by practitioners who have expertise in basic scientific inquiry. More typically, practitioners request an appropriate discipline to study the phenomena of concern. Working with members of the discipline, the practitioners tentatively identify the unknowns of the enigmatic problem. Once basic scientific inquiry begins, practitioners may direct the project, be among the participants, or may not be directly involved at all. Whatever their role, they follow the process closely, allowing themselves the opportunity for almost immediate access to the empirical data generated and to assess its suitability for dealing with the problem in question.

When the enigmatic problem is clear but appears intractable due to the lack of knowledge, turn attention to peripheral but associated problems.

Sets of guidelines for practice are developed for these problems. AIDS is a good example. Being unable to effectively control the HIV virus, sets of guidelines are being developed for dealing with opportunistic infections, other conditions associated with AIDS, and functional problems. A second example is the assistance given to individuals with spinal cord injuries. Since the spinal cord cannot be "repaired" with our current knowledge, sets of guidelines continue to be developed to resolve the multiple problems associated with spinal cord injuries.

Formulate an atheoretical set of guidelines using practical inquiry and folk knowledge.

Applied Type II inquiry is used to refine and assess the adequacy of the set of guidelines during and after its formulation. Atheoretical sets of guidelines should always be designated as such. Doing otherwise would be inaccurate, of course, but it would also inhibit further basic and applied Type I inquiry relative to the problem.

Accept the limits of our knowledge.

Some enigmatic problems cannot be dealt with because we do not know enough. No theories or empirical data provide sufficient direction—or even clues—as to how a problem might be resolved; pretending this is not so will only impede further knowing. But accepting effective, atheoretical sets of guidelines for which no theoretical support can be found is also difficult. Why do they work? How do they work? It is frustrating and disconcerting not to know.

Difficulties Associated with Sets of Guidelines for Practice

Any profession with a neopositivistic orientation is concerned about the current status, the overall adequacy, and the appropriate use of its collection of sets of guidelines for practice. The ever-changing nature of problem areas, theoretical knowledge, and professions themselves makes continual vigilance necessary. There are several general difficulties associated with sets of guidelines for practice.

The most obvious difficulty interfering with development of sets of guidelines for practice is the lack of knowledge about the process of doing so. Disagreement about what constitutes the "structure and required content" of a set of guidelines for practice specifically suited to the needs of a given profession contributes to this problem. In part, this situation may be due to uncertainty about what is an appropriate epistemological orientation for the profession, or there may be insufficient understanding of applied scientific inquiry.

A clearly stated domain of concern by a profession facilitates development of sets of guidelines. However, regardless of their clarity, domains of concern present their own problems. The taxonomy of a profession's domain of concern typically provides only one perspective regarding possible problem areas, only one way of perceiving and organizing information. A single perspective interferes with entertaining other ways of conceptualizing problems and of thinking about clients, the difficulties they might have, and their situations. Although no easy task, adopting a different perspective often prompts the identification of different problems and the development of new sets of guidelines for practice.

Professions are also hesitant to move outside the boundaries of their domains of concern. Enigmatic problems identified that could possibly be dealt with by the profession may not be considered because they are seen as only tangential to the profession's domain of concern. Such thinking limits exploration and, ultimately, is detrimental to assisting clients.

Third, a profession's domain of concern limits its views about problems leading to a belief that certain problems are not amenable to resolution. Thus, nothing is done. No attempt is made to develop sets of guidelines for practice. On the other hand, the profession may not recognize some problem areas. If the problems are not seen, they do not exist for the profession. A set of guidelines for practice cannot be developed until a problem is recognized.

The final difficulty related to the domain of concern is whether it accurately reflects a profession's expertise. There may be no sets of guidelines for practice for some elements of the domain of concern, or sets of guidelines for particular elements may be so obviously inadequate that their use is highly questionable. A profession must either develop new or more adequate sets of guidelines for these elements or must seriously consider whether the elements in question should remain part of the profession's domain of concern. The credibility of a profession is questioned when it claims that it can identify or resolve a problem when it really cannot do so.

Several issues related to theoretical information also present difficulties when creating sets of guidelines for practice. Often, atheoretical sets of guidelines are treated as if they were theoretically based because their lack of theoretical foundation may be unknown or ignored. Such guidelines are not studied to determine whether theoretical support is available, nor is the development of appropriate new theoretical knowledge sought. Atheoretical sets of guidelines are not uncommon in the health professions. The Bobaths' set of guidelines for practice is one example (Bobath, 1979). Atheoretical sets of guidelines are acceptable, however, only when recognized as such and when appropriate effort is directed towards seeking a theoretically sound foundation.

As has been mentioned, one of the complaints disciplines direct toward professions is that they use outdated theories and empirical data. Therefore, professions must continually assess their sets of guidelines to see that they are founded on the most current, valid theoretical information.

Professions ignore theories and empirical data that could be, and perhaps should be, used as the foundation for sets of guidelines for practice. This may be due in part to the general discomfort with theory. One consequence of this discomfort is failure to read and examine theoretical information. Only through the continual review of the literature of disciplines are professions able to keep informed about emerging, new, and revised theoretical information. One could go so far as to say that not using suitable theories and empirical data as the basis for developing or revising sets of guidelines is morally indefensible. How many lives would have been saved if Fleming's report on penicillin had been "noticed" when it was published in 1928 rather than being left unheeded until 1940?

Other areas of difficulty associated with sets of guidelines for practice appear in the final step in their development—consideration of internal consistency and completeness of content. In some sets of guidelines, the theories and empirical data used as the theoretical foundation do not consistently support the guidelines for problem identification and problem resolution. In other words, the guidelines seem to have been deduced from out of nowhere. At other times, the suggested evaluation procedures are directed towards identifying problems that are not adequately addressed in the guidelines for problem resolution. Or there may be guidelines for resolution of problems for which there are no guidelines for problem identification. In either case, there is not an adequate match between the areas evaluated and the focus of intervention.

Sets of guidelines for practice may be incomplete. The theoretical foundation may be suggested rather than specifically stated. Guidelines for problem identification or problem resolution may be too general or vague to be of any use, or some may be missing entirely. A series of case descriptions may be presented rather than guidelines for problem resolution. Although case descriptions are informative, they cannot be used as substitutes for guidelines for problem resolution.

An inadequate amount of Type II inquiry of sets of guidelines for practice is a chronic problem in most, if not all, health professions, particularly in relation to assessments of effectiveness. Multiple methodological and ethical issues are inherent in evaluative research, making such research complicated. But beyond that, there are entrenched practices and beliefs that limit evaluative research. For instance, professions use sets of guidelines that have been demonstrated to be ineffective, even though they know the guidelines are relatively useless. A conspiracy of silence arises regarding their inadequacy that, in turn, leads to a fear of assessing the adequacy of other sets of guidelines.

The belief that a set of guidelines for practice is effective when there is no empirical evidence to support such a belief is perhaps even more detrimental to the profession than simply a lack of sufficient evaluation research. Firmly held beliefs about effectiveness inhibit interest in studying the effectiveness of all sets of guidelines.

Evaluative research may also be inhibited by practitioners' emotional attachment to sets of guidelines for practice. They neither want to assess the adequacy of a particular set of guidelines nor acknowledge any data that suggest "their" set of guidelines may not be as effective or efficient as they believe. There is some evidence that studies have been inhibited regarding long-term effectiveness, for example, in occupational therapy relative to the sensory integration frame of reference (Ayres, 1979) and in medicine relative to coronary bypass surgery. Projects designed to gather information about adequacy may be severely criticized, as may be the investigator. Negative findings may even be repressed through the rejection of controversial research reports for publication.

Finally, sets of guidelines claimed by a profession to be used to deal with particular problems may not be precisely adhered to or may actually not be used at all. Practitioners may be using another set of guidelines or no discernable guidelines of any kind. Sets of guidelines for practice that are repeatedly misused or are not regularly followed need to be reassessed. Both applied Type I and Type II inquiry should be considered.

This listing of difficulties associated with sets of guidelines for practice is not meant to discourage readers; rather, its purpose is to point out possible problems in order to encourage and facilitate ongoing, honest examination of sets of guidelines for practice.

In so doing, a profession remains viable and able to effectively serve the society to which it is responsible.

11. Sets of Guidelines for Practice in Occupational Therapy

The information presented in Chapter 10 was concerned with sets of guidelines for practice in general. In order to describe the process of formulating sets of guidelines in more detail, this chapter examines sets of guidelines in one profession, occupational therapy. This is done for illustrative purposes only and is not meant to imply that the structure and content of sets of guidelines for practice in occupational therapy are appropriate for other professions.

The first section of the chapter deals with developing frames of reference, the set of guidelines for practice of occupational therapy. Primary attention is given to applied Type I inquiry. Although there are a few additional comments regarding applied Type II inquiry as it relates to multiple-component sets of guidelines for practice, on the whole, applied Type II inquiry seems to be the same irrespective of profession.

Frames of reference were originally designed to provide theoretically based sets of guidelines for practice for that aspect of occupational therapy intervention concerned with change—that is, development or restoration of function to the highest possible level. Their suitability for other aspects of intervention in occupational therapy—prevention, meeting universal needs, maintenance, and management—is questionable. The second section of the chapter is devoted to discussion of this issue of limited suitability, which is probably not exclusive to the profession of occupational therapy. The structure and requisite content of the typical set of guidelines of other professions may also not be suitable for all aspects of their practice.

Developing Frames of Reference

Before reading this section, the reader should review the description of frames of reference in Chapter 4 (pages 84-87). The discussion that follows builds on that description and on information presented in Chapter 10.

Specific structural issues related to developing frames of reference are emphasized in the following discussion. Practitioners usually have some idea of the theoretical information that is fundamental to change in many areas of the profession's domain of concern. However, they often have difficulty taking that information and putting it into the form of a frame of reference. Paying attention to structure may minimize this problem. As the majority of current frames of reference consist of multiple components, the following discussion focuses on developing such frames of reference (Mosey, 1981, 1986).

Theoretical Base

The theoretical base of a frame of reference is a collection of internally consistent concepts, definitions, and postulates derived from theoretical information that describes one or more elements of the profession's domain of concern and that provides information fundamental to identifying function and dysfunction and to enhancing function and/or minimizing dysfunction. The structure and content of frames of reference are illustrated schematically in Figure 9, which is used extensively in the following discussion.

The process of developing a frame of reference begins with analysis of an enigmatic problem. This should be done carefully and in depth as was described in the last chapter. In the next step, identification of suitable theories and empirical data, only primary sources are used. Information is not drawn from sets of guidelines for practice of other professions (e.g., "theories of instruction" or "behavioral modification") nor from texts that provide summaries or syntheses of various theories and empirical data. As

Figure 9. Content and structure of a frame of reference.

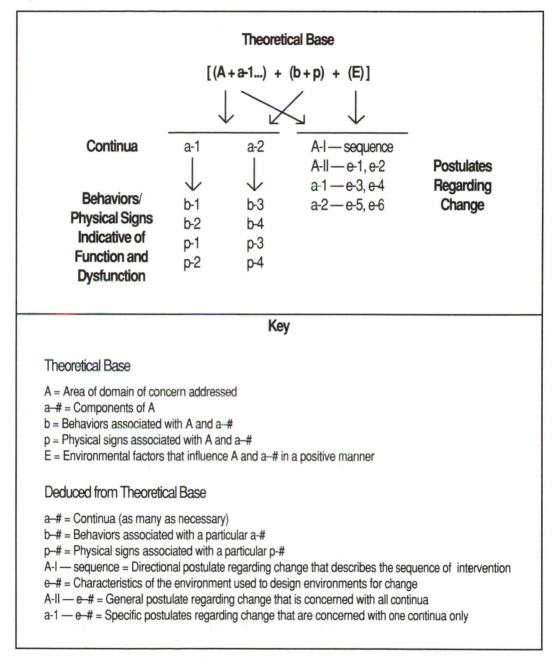

Theoretical Base

$$[(A + a\text{-}1...) + (b + p) + (E)]$$

Continua	a-1	a-2	A-I — sequence	
			A-II — e-1, e-2	**Postulates**
			a-1 — e-3, e-4	**Regarding**
Behaviors/	b-1	b-3	a-2 — e-5, e-6	**Change**
Physical Signs	b-2	b-4		
Indicative of	p-1	p-3		
Function and	p-2	p-4		
Dysfunction				

Key

Theoretical Base

A = Area of domain of concern addressed
a–# = Components of A
b = Behaviors associated with A and a–#
p = Physical signs associated with A and a–#
E = Environmental factors that influence A and a–# in a positive manner

Deduced from Theoretical Base

a–# = Continua (as many as necessary)
b–# = Behaviors associated with a particular a-#
p–# = Physical signs associated with a particular p-#
A-I — sequence = Directional postulate regarding change that describes the sequence of intervention
e–# = Characteristics of the environment used to design environments for change
A-II — e–# = General postulate regarding change that is concerned with all continua
a-1 — e–# = Specific postulates regarding change that are concerned with one continua only

Figure 9 shows, the practitioner seeks information about:

1. The area to be addressed in the frame of reference [A].

2. Components of the area to be addressed [a-1, a-2, a-3, etc.].

3. Behaviors [b] and physical signs [p], if any, associated with the area addressed and its components.

4. Environmental factors, both human and non-human, that influence the area addressed and its components in a positive manner [E].

A practical way of dealing with the collected information at this point is simply to list potentially useful postulates. The next step is to organize the postulates into three groups:

1. Description of the problem [A + a-1...].
2. Associated behaviors and physical signs [b + p].
3. Environmental factors [E].

For each group, all concepts are defined; redundant and superfluous concepts and postulates discarded; similar concepts combined and "new" concepts defined and labeled; and superordinate and subordinate conceptual levels identified. The need for additional information becomes apparent at various points in this process.

Next, the selected postulates are combined into an integrated whole. The ideal structure for a theoretical base is similar to that of an adequately structured theory (Chapter 8), but such a structure is likely only when a frame of reference is based on a single theory. Since frames of reference are usually founded on more than one theory and/or several pieces of empirical data, the structure of a theoretical base usually looks more like that illustrated in Figure 10.

The illustration is somewhat truncated; each of the groups stands for all of the information included in the theoretical description of it: the area addressed [A, a-1, etc.], behaviors associated with the area [b-1, b-2, etc.], physical signs associated with the area [p-1, p-2, etc.], and environmental factors likely to influence the area addressed in a positive manner [E, e-1, etc.]. Only theoretical information is included, not (a) ideas or suggestions about the application of information nor (b) reports of research findings regarding the information.

The solid lines connecting the area addressed with behavior and physical signs and with environmental factors represent postulates stating the relationships

Figure 10. Pictorial representation of the structure and content of the theoretical base of a frame of reference.

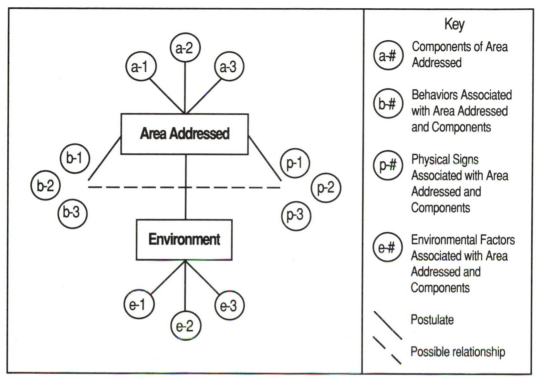

between these areas. There are no postulates stating the relationships between behaviors and physical signs and environmental factors because, on a theoretical level, intervention is not directed toward behaviors and physical signs but rather toward the problem addressed. There may or may not be a relationship between behaviors and physical signs represented by the broken line.

Adequate definitions of the area addressed and its components are essential. The components are carefully defined so as to be relatively mutually exclusive so that they may serve their intended purpose—forming the function/dysfunction continuum of the frame of reference. In other words, components must be sufficiently different from each other so that (a) there is little overlap in behaviors and physical signs used for problem identification and (b) each component can be dealt with separately in problem resolution. "Relative" is used to emphasize that any problem or problem component, no matter how small, is related to the entire functioning of the individual.

Components are defined so that they are on the same conceptual level. A component that is superordinate or subordinate to another component will ultimately lead to confusion. For instance, "coping skills" and "time management" are not equivalent components (nor are they mutually exclusive) because time management is considered to be part of coping skills and, thus, subordinate. Difficulties with nonequivalent conceptual levels and lack of exclusivity are closely related. When components are not adequately defined, the associated behaviors/physical signs indicative of function and dysfunction are likely to seem to come from nowhere. Moreover, content validity and the discreteness of the components (continua) will be difficult to establish when refining evaluation procedures.

A few comments on what kinds of theoretical information are suitable for use as a foundation for frames of reference. Because occupational therapy is concerned with designing environments to facilitate change, theoretical information is sought that describes how the environment (both human and nonhuman) can enhance function and how such an environment could be arranged.

Theoretical information made up of simple concepts is often more useful than information presented primarily in the form of constructs. Thus, theoretical information using hypothetical structures and mechanisms as a means of explanation should be avoided if at all possible. Information in this form is not sufficiently concrete to use as the basis for either problem identification or problem resolution. Theoretical information in the form of analogies, such as computer models of cognitive function, should also be avoided.

Finally, occupational therapy focuses on problem resolution through changes in behavior that are best described as learning. At least 80% of the profession's frames of reference are to some extent based on postulates selected from one or more theories of learning. Thus, when looking for suitable theoretical information relative to an enigmatic problem—particularly dynamic information—it may be helpful to survey various theories of learning.

Function-Dysfunction Continua

The function-dysfunction continua of a frame of reference are the components of the area of human function addressed in the frame of reference, a-1 and a-2 in Figure 9. Because the continua have been labeled and defined as such in the theoretical base, they are identified in this part of the frame of reference simply by the neutral label—such as "muscle strength" or "memory"—that they were assigned. The idea of a continuum—a range from functional to dysfunctional—need not be reflected in the label.

Some frames of reference conceptualize various areas of human function as developing in a stage-specific manner, such as grasping or the ability to interact in various types of groups. When this is the case, each stage is identified as a separate continuum. Although stages of development are not really discrete entities, evaluation is facilitated by treating each stage separately.

Behaviors and Physical Signs Indicative of Function and Dysfunction

Behaviors and physical signs indicative of function and dysfunction are the guidelines for problem identification in frames of reference. They are enumerated so as to be specific to each continuum and are used as the basis for evaluation (b-1, b-2, p-1, etc., in Figure 9). It should be noted that many frames of reference do not include physical signs. Behaviors/physical signs may be stated in a positive way, indicating adequate function (e.g., the individual is able to...); in a negative way, indicating dysfunction (e.g., the individual is not able to ...); or both. When only one indicator is presented, whether an indicator of function or dysfunction, it should be clearly stated that the absence of that indicator is evidence of its opposite—that is, the absence of a behavior that indicates function is evidence of dysfunction.

In Figure 9, behaviors and physical signs are listed for each of the continua. They could be indicative of function, dysfunction, or a combination of both. The numerals in the symbols—b-1, b-2, p-1, p-2, etc.—are used to highlight the idea that behaviors and physical signs are specific to a continuum. Thus, b-1 and p-1 are used for only one continuum, a-1. Accurate and discriminate problem identification can only take place when there is minimal or no overlap between the behaviors/physical signs for each of the continua included in the frame of reference. The number of behaviors and physical signs listed for each continuum should be sufficient for problem identification—no more and no less. In other words, if three behaviors/ physical signs are sufficient for problem identification, there is no need to list additional behaviors/ physical signs for that continuum.

Behaviors indicative of function and dysfunction are stated in such a way that they are able to serve as the conceptual framework for activity analysis and synthesis relative to designing evaluation situations or procedures. Activities are analyzed to determine their potential for eliciting the behaviors indicative of function and dysfunction as enumerated in a given frame of reference. For example, if a behavior indicative of function is stated as "comfortable in unstructured situations," activities would be analyzed relative to whether or not they provide structure.

Activities for evaluation are synthesized based on knowledge of the collection of behaviors the practitioner will need to observe for problem identification. Ideally, each of the activities selected for evaluation elicits more than one of the behaviors that need to be observed, thus making the process more efficient. Nevertheless, the evaluation activities as a group must also allow the practitioner to differentiate between each continuum and, when appropriate, level or degree of function. From these processes, more formal or standardized evaluative procedures are developed, if that is deemed desirable.

Postulates Regarding Change

Postulates regarding change are the guidelines for problem resolution in frames of reference. Figure 9 illustrates the three types:

1. A directional postulate, A-I—sequence.

This postulate provides precepts regarding where to begin the process of problem resolution relative to the various components and what the recommended sequence of the change process should be. A directional postulate is stated only when the change process would be enhanced by addressing the components in a specific sequence of intervention.

2. A general postulate regarding change, A-II—e-1, e-2.

A general postulate, applicable to all continua,

describes those environmental factors [e-1, e-2] considered to be essential for resolution of the problem addressed. For example, when a frame of reference concerned with activities of daily living is based on Bandura's learning theory (1977), a general postulate might describe how people will act as models and how imitation of these models will be fostered. A general postulate is not included when there are no environmental factors common to problem resolution for all continua.

3. A specific postulate, represented by a-1—e-3, e-4, and a-2—e-5, e-6.

Specific postulates provide guidelines for problem resolution for each of the continua in the frame of reference. They describe the characteristics of the environment—including the actions of the practitioner—that are needed to foster change. Only the properties of activities are identified, rather than specific activities. Particular activities may be mentioned, however, for the purpose of clarification. Specific postulates do not describe what the client will or will not do in some unspecified manner. For example, this specific postulate regarding change describes the characteristics of the environment: "The ability to organize a task is enhanced through engaging in activities that cannot be successfully completed without adequate organization by the task participant; such activities are graded according to the degree of organization required, the number of steps, the tools and materials needed, and the time required to complete." Contrast this with a postulate describing what a client will do: "The ability to organize a task is enhanced through learning how to think about a task prior to engaging in it." Notice that no information about how to design an environment to enhance the ability to organize a task is provided.

General and specific postulates regarding change usually have these formal characteristics:

1. The label for the area addressed in the frame of reference (for a general postulate) or for the continuum (for specific postulates).

2. A bridging term such as "is enhanced through" or "facilitated by."

3. A listing of the appropriate environmental factors.

General and specific postulates regarding change serve as the conceptual framework for analyzing and synthesizing activities that can be used to enhance function. Activities are analyzed according to what degree they have the characteristics stated in the various postulates regarding change. Thus, returning to the last example regarding the ability to organize a task, activities would be analyzed according to the level of organization they would require.

Activities are synthesized to be as compatible as possible with the entire postulate. In other words, based on the analysis, activities are selected, designed, or manipulated in such a way that they provide the environmental characteristics required for problem resolution. The interests and values of the client are always taken into consideration in activity synthesis.

Activity analysis and synthesis for problem identification should not be confused with analysis and synthesis for problem resolution. Not only is the purpose different, but so are the activity characteristics that need to be identified. In evaluation with a client, one is concerned only with eliciting a sufficient sample of behavior to determine whether or not there is a problem. In intervention, eliciting behavior is often required, but one is concerned more with designing an environment that will foster change.

When all of the above has been accomplished, the frame of reference is ready for consideration of internal consistency and completeness of content as described in Chapter 10. Attention then shifts to refining and assessing the adequacy of the frame of reference using applied Type II inquiry.

Applied Type II inquiry is used to determine whether the components of the problem or the continua are truly different from each other—that is, whether they have differential validity. Often, investigators use factor analysis—a statistical method that, among other things, identifies to what extent data form clusters (Cronbach, 1985). Simply put, when the continua are appropriately discrete, evaluative findings (using the evaluative procedures that are part of the frame of reference) should cluster around each of the identified continua. When the predicted clusters are not found, the continua need to be reexamined because some of them may not be sufficiently mutually exclusive to warrant treating them as separate components. However, the clusters that do form in the factor analysis may provide information about how the components might be reformulated.

Factor analysis is also a useful method for refining evaluation procedures employed in sets of guidelines for practice in which a problem is treated as a single entity. It may highlight evaluation data that are not needed for definitive problem identification. The evaluation procedure can then be revised so as to avoid collecting irrelevant or redundant data, resulting in greater efficiency. On the other hand, if more than one cluster of data is found, the sets of guidelines may not be focused on a single problem but rather on one made up of two or more components.

Other Types of Sets of Guidelines for Practice

The structure and requisite content of frames of reference provide guidelines for the change process—that is, the development or restoration of function to the highest possible level. More specifically, therapists and clients anticipate and work toward significant alteration in the clients' ability to function. Change, whether direct or compensatory in nature, is considered to be located within the client. Altering the environment to enable a client to function more comfortably and effectively is not considered change; it is maintenance. When the design of such an environment involves physical alteration, whether it be the addition of a simple piece of equipment or a complex electronic system, it is based on technological guidelines and is not part of the change process per se. However, learning how to use and interact within an environment that has been altered *is* part of the change process.

Because frames of reference are oriented to the change process, they are not suitable as a set of guidelines for the other aspects of occupational therapy practice—prevention, meeting universal needs, maintenance, and management. Therefore, if the profession is to have adequate sets of guidelines for practice, either (a) the structure and required content of frames of reference must be altered so as to accommodate the other aspects of practice or (b) additional types of sets of guidelines need to be created.

The author has tried to alter frames of reference to accommodate other aspects of practice with no success. In all attempts, the specified structure and required content had to be so broadly stated that there was insufficient direction for engaging in applied Type I inquiry. More significantly, the resulting sets of guidelines for practice were so vague that they did not provide adequate direction for either problem identification or problem resolution.

If the need for additional types of sets of guidelines for practice is clear, exactly what they should look like is problematic. The occupational therapy literature describes various programs designed for prevention, meeting universal needs, maintenance, and management, but there are no discernable patterns of "necessary structure and content" to serve as the basis for creating sets of guidelines for practice for each of these various aspects of practice. The exception is the work of Claudia Allen (1985) regarding maintenance, which will be discussed later.

What follows, then, is a brief outline of the possible "necessary structure and content" for a set of guidelines for practice for each aspect of practice other than the change process (Mosey, 1986).

Prevention Prevention is the process of facilitating function for individuals in areas where a potential for dysfunction exists, especially those individuals "at risk" for developing dysfunction. Prevention is different than maintenance, which is concerned with assisting individuals who already have some problems in functioning.

Sets of guidelines for practice directed towards prevention would need to contain the following information:

Theoretical foundation:
- The nature of the problem to be prevented.
- Behaviors on the part of the individual that are likely to prevent the problem from occurring and how such behaviors are acquired or promoted.
- Environmental factors (human and nonhuman)

that are likely to prevent the problem from occurring.

Guidelines for determining whether an individual is at risk:
- Behaviors that indicate a person is, or is likely to be, at risk for developing the problem.
- Environmental or personal situations that may lead to the development of the problem.

Guidelines for prevention:
- Principles to guide acquisition of new behavior or increasing the frequency of previously acquired behavior.
- Principles to guide environmental alteration.

Meeting Universal Needs

Meeting universal needs is the process of assisting others to satisfy the inherent human needs for physical, psychological, and social well-being that are shared by all people regardless of their present state of health, illness, or disability. Examples include the need for acceptance, the need to feel secure, and the need to control at least some aspects of one's life situation. Meeting universal needs is differentiated from the change process, which is concerned with assisting individuals to learn how to meet their own needs. Meeting universal needs does not involve skill acquisition; rather, it creates an environment in which needs are likely to be satisfied with minimal effort on the part of the individual. For example, practitoners may creating an environment where individuals feel accepted and safe by having sufficient personnel so that there are people close by in case assistance is needed, by providing a map of the area and an outline of the safety measures to be followed in the event of a fire, by placing call-bells in bedrooms and bathrooms, and by providing locked places for the clients' personal items.

Sets of guidelines for practice for meeting universal needs should include the following information:

Theoretical foundation:
- Description of a comprehensive system of universal needs and definitions of those needs.
- Description of environmental factors conducive to satisfying each identified need.

Guidelines for determining whether an individual's universal needs are currently being met:

- A list of the needs described in the theoretical foundation.
- Behaviors indicative of need satisfaction/lack of satisfaction for each of the listed needs.

Guidelines for meeting universal needs:
- Principles to guide creation of an environment conducive to satisfying each of the identified needs.

Maintenance   Maintenance is the process of preserving and supporting an individual's current level of function after appropriate efforts have been made to diminish dysfunction and enhance function. The level of maintenance often depends on the usual course of the condition: (a) little change over an extended period of time, assuming that adequate efforts are directed towards maintenance; (b) alternating periods of exacerbation and remission; or (c) an anticipated continued worsening of the condition.

In occupational therapy, two types of maintenance exist: one focuses on a circumscribed area to which a regimen of maintenance is directed, such as an arthritic condition; the other type is concerned with maintenance of an optimal level of function when a major deficit affects most areas of function, such as in Alzheimer's disease.

When maintenance is concerned with a *circumscribed area*, a set of guidelines for practice should include the following information:

Theoretical foundation:
- Definition and description of the area addressed, including the typical course.
- Biological, behavioral, and environmental factors positively influencing maintenance.
- Factors influencing learning and compliance with a prescribed regimen.

Guidelines for determining the extent and type of maintenance required:
- Some type of taxonomy that allows for delineation of current status—for instance, stages, phases, or degree of severity.
- Behavior and physical signs that indicate current status relative to course.

Guidelines for maintenance in a circumscribed area:
- Principles for developing a regimen of maintenance relating to the categories in the defined taxonomy.
- Principles to guide teaching the regimen to the client and increasing the probability of compliance.

Allen's work (1985) is oriented to the second type of maintenance—maintaining an optimal level of function when a major deficit affects most areas of function. Allen developed an evaluation tool designed to identify levels of functioning of individuals with general cognitive deficits regardless of diagnosis. The purpose of the tool is to determine whether an individual is in need of a protected environment and, if so, the degree or level of protection that will be required. Allen also described environmental characteristics that would ensure adequate protection of individuals with various degrees of cognitive dysfunction.

Following Allen's work, a set of guidelines for practice concerned with maintenance when there is a *major deficit* should include the following information:

Theoretical foundation:
- Definition and description of the area of major loss and its impact on overall function.
- Levels of deficit severity.
- Environmental elements that allow for maximum satisfying function despite deficit.

Guidelines for determining levels of severity:
- Specified levels.
- Behaviors indicating ability to function at each level.

Guidelines for maintenance when there is a major deficit:
- Principles to guide creating an environment that fosters maximum and satisfying functioning at specified levels.

Management
Management is the process of minimizing a client's distressing or disruptive feelings and behaviors so that the client and the practitioner are able to deal more directly, effectively, and efficiently with primary problems. These feelings/behaviors may be immedi-

ately related to the primary problem, such as pain or confusion, or may be more general, as with general anxiety or denial. Since the concept of management is based on the assumption that distressing feelings/ behaviors will ultimately fade away as the primary problem is resolved, management is concerned with "in the meantime."

A set of guidelines for practice directed toward client management may be addressed to one or to a variety of distressing feelings/behaviors. What would be included in one set of guidelines depends upon the extent to which there is common theoretical support. The information needed for an adequate set of guidelines addressing one distressing feeling/behavior should include:

Theoretical foundation:
- Definition and description of the distressing feeling/behavior.
- Environmental factors considered to be related to the distressing feeling/behavior.

Guidelines for determining the presence of the distressing feelings/behavior:
- Behaviors that indicate the presence of the distressing feeling.
- Behaviors that differentiate the distressing feeling/behavior addressed from other feelings/ behavior (e.g., the difference between confusion and withdrawal).

Guidelines for management:
- Principles to guide creation of an environment that is likely to diminish the distressing feeling/behavior.

The extent to which occupational therapists are knowledgeable about and use theories and empirical data as the foundation for prevention, meeting universal needs, maintenance, and management seems to vary with the focus of practice. On the whole, prevention (fairly uncommon in occupational therapy) and maintenance appear to be based on theoretical information.

Meeting universal needs and management are often part of a total intervention process but are given little attention because they tend to be engaged in

Applied Scientific Inquiry in the Health Professions

outside of the therapist's acknowledged interventions. Little consideration has been given to the theoretical foundation for these aspects of practice. The therapist comforting a crying child would often be unable to describe theoretical support for the action taken. Much that is done to meet universal needs and management seems to be based on specific solutions. It is here that the past traditional epistemological orientation of the profession is most evident.

This section ends pretty much where it began. The question still remains whether frames of reference can or should be altered to accommodate all aspects of practice, or whether different types of sets of guidelines for practice are needed for each aspect of practice. The advantage of altering frames of reference to address all aspects of practice is that the profession would only need to deal with one type of sets of guideline for practice. With only one type of sets of guidelines for practice, there would be a loss of precision and specificity, however. A separate type of sets of guidelines for each aspect of practice may assist the profession in: (a) recognizing and differentiating between the five aspects of practice, (b) giving greater attention to the theoretical foundation for meeting universal needs and management, as well as the other aspects of practice, and (c) formulating more precise sets of guidelines for practice.

Section V:
Postprofessional Education

Much has been written about basic or entry-level professional education in the health professions. This may be due, in part, to both higher enrollment and to accreditation by professional organizations of programs at this level. Far less has been written about postprofessional education.

The following chapter focuses on postprofessional education for two reasons. First, the information presented may lead to more discussion about this level of education. Second, it is within postprofessional education that the need for a clearly stated epistemology of practice is most apparent. In Chapter 12, attention is given to: (a) a statement of a philosophy of postprofessional education, (b) differentiation of postprofessional education from other types of education, and (c) positions on various issues related to postprofessional education.

12. *Postprofessional Education within a Neopositivistic Orientation*

A profession's epistemological orientation exerts a strong influence on its philosophy of education. Consequently, a lack of a clear epistemological orientation often leads to uncertainty about the purpose and focus of education.

A philosophy of education is a collection of congruent beliefs and values that serve as a foundation for establishing educational objectives and priorities, identifying levels of instruction, and designing educational programs. The latter includes making decisions about content and processes to be taught, organization of material, methods of instruction, and means of assessing mastery. A profession's philosophy of education ultimately determines what knowledge, skills, and attitudes are necessary for clinicians and scholars to carry out the work of the profession in a competent manner.

The following discussion is presented from the viewpoint of the neopositivistic orientation. An epistemological orientation per se does not directly address educational issues, but what it does offer is a perspective for considering these issues and a context for formulating a philosophy of education. This involves inductive reasoning; thus, there is always the possibility of moving beyond the boundaries of a given epistemological orientation. On occasion, this may be the case in the following discussion.[1]

Definition and a Philosophy of Postprofessional Education

Postprofessional education is a course of study leading to a master's or doctoral degree that is offered by an academic department of professional studies for individuals who have completed entry-level education in that profession.

A philosophy of postprofessional education derived from the neopositivistic orientation is based on the following beliefs:

1. A health profession is responsible for the education of its members to ensure competent, ethical clinical practice.

2. A health profession is responsible for the education of a coterie of members who are skilled in doing the scholarly work of the profession, which includes examining, developing, refining, and evaluating the profession's (a) fundamental body of knowledge, (b) applied body of knowledge, and (c) practice.

3. A profession is responsible for the education of its clinical and academic educators.

The primary purpose of postprofessional education is to prepare individuals to do the scholarly work of the profession—that is, to engage in the applied scientific and philosophical inquiry necessary for the well-being of the profession. In terms of applied scientific inquiry, students are prepared to: (a) first, evaluate and refine current sets of guidelines for practice relative to the validity of their theoretical foundation, internal consistency, completeness of content, and ad-

---

[1] In part, the ideas presented below are drawn from the work of Brooks, 1988; Fleming, Johnson, Marina, Spergel, and Townson, 1987; Fox, 1986; Glazer, 1980; Goodlad, 1984; Hughes, 1973; Kerlinger, 1960; McGlothlin, 1964; Perutz, 1989; Rodgers, 1986; Rule, 1978; Schein, 1972; Thorne, 1973; and Wulff, Pedersen, and Rosenberg, 1986. Not all of the authors directly address postprofessional education in the health professions, nor are their ideas necessarily congruent with those presented here. Rather, they served as the beginning point for the ideas presented below.

equacy; and (b) second, develop, refine, and assess the adequacy of new sets of guidelines for practice. Moreover, they are prepared to identify any lack of theoretical information in specific areas fundamental to the practice of the profession. Concomitantly, students are assisted in learning how to initiate, form, and work within those profession-discipline relationships that facilitate profession-directed, problem-oriented basic scientific inquiry on the part of appropriate disciplines. The intent of these two foci is to enable graduates to contribute to fashioning and maintaining an applied body of knowledge so that it provides the foundation for adequate problem identification and resolution with clients in those areas that constitute the profession's domain of concern.

Third, students are prepared to identify questions about practice, education, the activities of the profession, and related matters that may be able to be addressed through applied Type II inquiry; to plan and initiate such inquiry; and to interpret the resulting findings.

With regard to philosophical inquiry, students are prepared to identify, investigate, and formulate statements about those philosophical issues of concern to the profession:

1. Beliefs, values, and goals of the profession (assumptions).
2. Ethical principles, standards, and behavior.
3. The art of practice.
4. Philosophy of applied scientific inquiry, including the epistemology of practice.
5. Priorities relative to applied scientific inquiry.
6. Focus and content of technical, professional, continuing, and postprofessional education.
7. Future goals and directions of the profession.
8. Public and private policies regarding the delivery of health services.

Mastery of philosophical inquiry enables graduates to identify and present philosophical issues to the profession in a way that encourages cognizant examination. Equipped with their skills, graduates may guide the profession in adequately reconciling or resolving the philosophical issues fundamental to the activities of the profession and its interactions with society.

Finally, students are prepared to use both applied scientific and philosophical inquiry for the purpose of maintaining congruence among the profession's fundamental body of knowledge (and the internal consistency of its five parts), applied body of knowledge, and practice. Although an ever-changing profession may have incongruities within and among its bodies of knowledge, these problems can be minimized by adequate scholarly attention. The ability to assist in maintaining some degree of congruence is acquired in postprofessional programs.

The preparation of competent clinical and academic educators is also the responsibility of a profession. How this is best accomplished is not clear. However, an apprentice relationship with a skilled educator is often considered to be an expedient and effective way of gaining beginning mastery in these roles. Preparation of competent educators may—but need not—take place within a postprofessional program. When part of a program, it is considered to be secondary to preparing individuals to do the scholarly work of the profession.

Differentiation from Other Educational Programs

One way of examining and clarifying postprofessional education is to contrast it with other types of educational programs. Four types are described here: professional, continuing, "alternative," and postdoctoral.

Professional Education

Professional education is an academically based course of study that prepares individuals for entry into a profession as full participants in the clinical work of the profession. The qualifier "full participants" distinguishes professional education from a course of study concerned with preparing individuals for entry into a profession as technicians or assistants. A question of concern in some professions is what is the appropriate academic level for professional education— baccalaureate or master's? While the author takes no position here, one of the tasks involved in making the decision is identifying the goals of professional education versus those of continuing and postprofessional education.

Professional education has two major objectives from the neopositivistic perspective. The first is to assist individuals in acquiring the knowledge, skills, and attitudes necessary for competent and ethical participation in clinical practice. To reach this objective, students are assisted in:

1. Gaining an understanding of the neopositivistic epistemological orientation to practice.

2. Mastering the profession's fundamental and applied bodies of knowledge.

3. Acquiring skill in selecting and using the profession's collective sets of guidelines for practice as the basis for problem identification and resolution with a broad spectrum of clients.

The organization of knowledge in a neopositivistic orientation brings specificity and order to what is to be learned. The fundamental body of knowledge, with its five categories of information, provides an outline for organizing the content of basic courses. Most of the knowledge necessary for directly assisting clients is specified in the profession's applied body of knowledge within the integrated "wholes" of sets of guidelines for practice. Sets of guidelines for practice also provide the core around which beginning skills in clinical reasoning and decision making are acquired and the art of practice is nurtured.

Education within the neopositivistic orientation emphasizes the relationship between theoretical knowledge and practice. Students are provided with a sound background in the nature of theory and given an opportunity to explore theories and empirical data in their original, complete forms, rather than through summaries or syntheses of information. Students are taught the specific postulates that provide theoretical support for each set of guidelines for practice, not just given vague generalities like "kinesiology" or "group process." In studying the profession's various sets of guidelines for practice, findings from applied Type II inquiry are emphasized regarding the reliability and validity of problem identification and the safety, effectiveness, efficiency and acceptability to clients of the guidelines.

The second major objective of professional education is to introduce students to the scholarly activities that support the profession: applied scientific inquiry and philosophical inquiry. A student learns about what is involved in applied scientific and philosophical inquiry, as opposed to developing in-depth knowledge and skills for engaging in such investigation. Students are introduced to the methods of science and given an overview of the processes involved in developing, refining, and assessing the adequacy of sets of guidelines for practice. A beginning understanding of philosophical inquiry is gained through the consideration of the profession's philosophical assumptions and code of ethics, which involves examining the origin and nature of these parts of the profession's fundamental body of knowledge and their influence on daily practice.

Continuing Education

Continuing education is any activity engaged in subsequent to professional education that enhances one's professional knowledge and skill, except courses of study leading to an academic degree. This is a broad definition and includes such activities as reading books and journals; attending conferences, inservice programs, and workshops; being involved in special interest and study groups; taking individual courses, academic or otherwise; having informal apprenticeships with master clinicians; and participating in long-term, clinically based and oriented programs subsequent to professional education (such as those available for physicians).

Although the goals may vary, by far the majority of continuing education experiences seek to enhance clinical knowledge and skills in specialized areas, with particular populations, or in nontraditional settings. Emphasis is often on keeping informed about and learning to use new or emerging sets of guidelines for practice and on gaining understanding of their underlying theoretical bases. Continuing educational experiences also may be directed toward parapractice areas, such as supervision, consultation, administration, and health planning and policy making.

The importance of continuing education for individuals and professions cannot be over emphasized. It is often only through such experiences that practitioners are able to maintain and increase their competence as clinicians and in parapractice areas. However, only rarely is continuing education directed toward developing the knowledge and skills necessary for scholarly pursuits. Such development usually takes place in an academic setting through postprofessional education. Besides tradition, the primary reasons for this are the availability of educators with expertise in scholarly pursuits and the length of time it takes to master the requisite knowledge and skills.

"Alternative" Education

Alternative education refers to a degree program— one that is located in an academic department other than that of an individual's professional education— taken subsequent to completion of professional education. While there are various reasons for participating in such programs, the primary ones are:

1. To augment clinical knowledge and skills by participating in programs of professions other than one's own, such as an occupational therapist participating in an entry-level program in special education.

2. To enhance parapractice knowledge and skills by participating in programs such as those offered by schools of public health or health administration.

3. To gain greater theoretical knowledge in a particular area and/or to acquire skill in conducting basic scientific inquiry by participating in degree programs offered by one of the disciplines.

Unlike postprofessional education, alternative education is not concerned with developing knowledge and skills fundamental to the scholarly work of professions.

Postdoctoral Professional Education

Postdoctoral professional education is formal, planned courses of study taken under the supervision of recognized scholars for the purpose of further enhancing scholarly knowledge and skills initially gained through postprofessional doctoral study. Although the goal may be to enhance scholarly knowledge and skills in general, more typically postdoctoral professional education is highly specialized, focusing on investigation in a limited area of a profession's fundamental or applied body of knowledge.

Postdoctoral professional education is distinguished from postprofessional education in that the latter is concerned with developing basic scholarly knowledge and skills applicable to many areas of the profession's bodies of knowledge. Postprofessional education serves as the foundation for postdoctoral professional education; alternative education does not provide such a foundation.

Positions on Related Issues

The following issues seem to be raised most often in discussions about postprofessional education: (a) the relationship between professional and postprofessional education, (b) the relationship between postprofessional master's and doctoral programs, (c) clinical specialization, (d) parapractice roles, (e) instruction in scientific inquiry, and (f) content versus process. The position taken on these issues is from a neopositivistic perspective, based on the educational philosophy outlined above and drawn from the author's experience.

Relationship between Professional and Postprofessional Education

Postprofessional programs are viewed as distinct from professional programs. An opposing position is that postprofessional master's programs (but usually not doctoral programs) are a fairly direct extension of professional education. Proponents of the latter position believe master's programs should instruct students in greater depth about subjects that were taught, or should have been taught, at the professional level.

As indicated earlier, professional programs are primarily designed to prepare students to be practitioners—that is, to become skilled in the clinical work of the profession. Although students should be given an understanding of the scholarly work of the profession, this is secondary to the task of becoming a clinician. Postprofessional study, on the other hand, is oriented to developing knowledge, skills, and attitudes fundamental to doing the scholarly work of the profession. Postprofessional programs should not be designed to make up for deficits in professional education.

Relationship between Postprofessional Master's and Doctoral Programs

Postprofessional master's and doctoral programs are viewed as part of a continuum of education in which master's programs are designed to be the first step toward a doctoral degree. Master's programs are similar to doctoral study, differing only in breadth and depth but not focus. The line between the two levels of education depends on the particular program and how a given student organizes his or her course of study. Nevertheless, postprofessional master's programs may be designed to be self-contained, terminal-degree experiences—that is, the course of study is complete unto itself.

In most health professions today, in which only a few individuals complete doctoral studies, the scholarly work of a profession cannot be left to these select few but must be carried out by others. Thus, master's programs are designed to prepare practitioners for this work, albeit at a less sophisticated level. In addition, individuals who participate in "preparatory" master's programs seem to be more likely to continue on to doctoral study than individuals in programs not seen as part of a master's-doctoral continuum. This master's-doctoral continuum is assumed in discussion of the remaining issues.

Clinical Specialization

From the neopositivistic perspective, postprofessional programs are not concerned with areas of clinical specialization or the education of master clinicians. Traditionally, universities have not been in the business of educating practitioners as practitioners beyond the professional level of preparation (Gurin & Williams, 1973; Hughes, 1973). Universities have usually seen their role in postprofessional education as preparing individuals to contribute to the body of knowledge of their profession.

The knowledge and skills necessary for becoming a master clinician are probably best acquired in a clinically based continuing education program with a strong apprenticeship component. Clinical skills cannot be taught in a classroom. Although one must learn about new and emerging theoretical information and sets of guidelines for practice in order to become a master clinician, there is no reason why such content cannot be taught in a program of continuing education and in the context of acquiring clinical skills.

In many health professions, the lines between various areas of clinical specialization are not clear relative to problem areas, theoretical information, sets of guidelines for practice used, issues of concern, or population. Because knowledge and skills are not particular to any area of specialization, thinking in terms of specialization may not be a constructive way of conceptualizing postprofessional education. It may be more fruitful to organize postprofessional programs around the knowledge and skills necessary for carrying out the scholarly work of the profession, rather than around areas of specialization.

Finally, when an attempt is made to combine the areas of clinical specialization and acquisition of scholarly skills, there is a tendency to give more attention to clinical specialization than to scholarly skills. Both students and faculty are inclined to drift toward issues directly related to practice because of the concrete and tangible qualities of such issues. It is more difficult to sustain the abstract thinking necessary for mastery of scholarly skills.

Parapractice Roles

Parapractice roles—supervision, administration, consultation, and health planning and policy making—are not particular to any clinically focused or "practice" health profession. Although practice professions draw upon the applied bodies of knowledge of these areas, on the whole they do not see contributing to these bodies of knowledge as their responsibility. Thus, the legitimacy of practice professions providing postprofessional programs or courses in these areas is difficult to support. This is not to deny the importance of parapractice roles. However, practitioners interested in pursuing study in these areas are best advised to participate in appropriate continuing education experiences or to seek admission into academic programs offered by departments of health administration and public health.

Instruction in Scientific Inquiry

Instruction in applied scientific inquiry, as opposed to basic inquiry, is given priority in postprofessional education. Although attention is given to research designs, emphasis is placed on the nature and methods of scientific inquiry. In other words, research designs are presented as only tools used in scientific inquiry. Study of research designs should not be seen as a substitute for the study of scientific inquiry. Sufficient instruction is given in basic scientific inquiry to enable students: (a) to engage in applied Type I inquiry, (b) to understand the various relationships between basic and applied scientific inquiry, and (c) to take a leadership role in those profession-discipline relationships concerned with problem-oriented basic inquiry.

Process versus Content

"Process" refers to a systematic series of intellectual activities by which an end is attained. "Content" refers to subjects, topics, or circumscribed sets of information. Reasoning, analysis, and interpretation are processes; theories, sets of guidelines for practice, and ethical principles are content.

Mastery of content—and content alone—is typical of continuing education. Postprofession education, on the other hand, is primarily concerned with process. The scholarly work of a profession is carried out through the various combinations of processes recognized as being fundamental to both scientific and philosophical inquiry. In this text, these processes have been referred to as the "methods of science" (see Chapter 7). The "methods of philosophy" are the same. The difference between scientific inquiry and philosophical inquiry is primarily in the phenomena addressed and the goals, not in the methods or processes used.

Only a few students come to postprofessional education with skill in using the methods of scholarly inquiry (process). Moreover, because mastery of process rarely occurs automatically with content learning, direct instruction in process needs to be a major part of postprofessional education. At least some courses should be specifically designed to teach process. Since mastery of process takes considerable time, these courses should not emphasize acquisition of content. If the pressure to learn content is minimized, more time is left to explore and master process. When a course is designed to teach relatively equal amounts of process and content, the majority of time usually ends up being devoted to content.

Process should also be emphasized in post-professional education because the theoretical information, sets of guidelines for practice, and philosophical issues of today may well be irrelevant in the near future. Content should be used primarily as a vehicle for learning process—for learning how to do the scholarly work of a profession.

In conclusion, postprofessional education is strongly influenced by a profession's epistemology of practice, and it is enhanced by a clearly defined orientation. It is within postprofessional education programs that a profession prepares practitioners to become the scientists and philosophers responsible for leading the profession into the future.

Appendices:
A Brief Outline of Occupational Therapy's Fundamental Body of Knowledge

A: Philosophical Assumptions

The philosophical assumptions of occupational therapy are the profession's basic beliefs about the nature of the individual and the environment, about the relationship between the individual and the environment, and about the proposes and goals of the profession relative to meeting the needs of the society. Distilled from the literature of the profession, these assumptions are:

1. Each individual has a right to a meaningful existence; to live in surroundings that are safe, supportive, comfortable, and over which he or she has some control; to make decisions for him or herself; to be productive; to experience pleasure and joy; and to love and be loved.

2. Each individual is influenced by the biological and social nature of the species.

3. Each individual can only be understood within the context of his or her family, friends, community, and cultural group membership.

4. Each individual has the need to participate in a variety of social roles and to have periodic relief from participation.

5. Each individual has the right to seek his or her potential through personal choice, within the context of accepted social constraints.

6. Each individual is able to reach his of her potential through purposeful interaction with the human and nonhuman environment.

7. Occupational therapy is concerned with promoting functional interdependence through in-

teractions directed toward facilitating participation in major social roles (areas of occupational performance) and with developing the sensorimotor, cognitive, psychological, and social components (performance components) fundamental to such roles.

8. The extent to which intervention is focused either on areas of occupational performance or on performance components is dependent upon the needs of a particular individual at any given time.

B: *Code of Ethics*

The code of ethics of occupational therapy consists of rules of conduct that describe practitioners' rights, obligations, and prohibited activities relative to others (clients, society, students, and colleagues), as well as principles of human conduct that serve as a guide for determining what is moral behavior in practice, parapractice activities, education, and research.

As published by the American Occupational Therapy Association (1988), the profession's code of ethics is:

Occupational Therapy Code of Ethics[1]

The American Occupational Therapy Association and its component members are committed to furthering people's ability to function fully within their total environment. To this end the occupational therapist renders service to clients in all stages of health and illness, to institutions, to other professionals and colleagues, to students, and to the general public.

In furthering this commitment, the American Occupational Therapy Association has established the Occupational Therapy Code of Ethics. This code is intended to be used as a guide to promoting and maintaining the highest standards of ethical behavior.

This Code of Ethics shall apply to all occupational therapy personnel. The term "occupational therapy personnel" shall include individuals who are regis-

---

[1] This document was approved by the Representative Assembly in April 1988; it replaces the (1977/1979) "Principles of Occupational Therapy Ethics." Reprinted with permission of the author.

tered occupational therapists, certified occupational therapy assistants, and occupational therapy students. The roles of practitioner, educator, manager, researcher, and consultant are assumed.

Principle 1 (Beneficence/ Autonomy) Occupational therapy personnel shall demonstrate a concern for the welfare and dignity of the recipient of their services.

    A. The individual is responsible for providing services without regard to race, creed, national origin, sex, age, handicap, disease entity, social status, financial status, or religious affiliation.

    B. The individual shall inform those people served of the nature and potential outcomes of treatment and shall respect the right of potential recipients of service to refuse treatment.

    C. The individual shall inform subjects involved in education or research activities of the potential outcome of those activities.

    D. The individual shall include those people served in the treatment planning process.

    E. The individual shall maintain goal-directed and objective relationships with all people served.

    F. The individual shall protect the confidential nature of information gained in educational, practice, and investigational activities unless sharing such information could be deemed necessary to protect the well-being of a third party.

    G. The individual shall take all reasonable precautions to avoid harm to the recipient of services or detriment to the recipient's property.

    H. The individual shall establish fees, based on cost analysis, that are commensurate with services rendered.

Principle 2 (Competence) Occupational therapy personnel shall actively maintain high standards of professional competence.

    A. The individual shall hold the appropriate credential for providing service.

    B. The individual shall recognize the need for competence and shall participate in continuing professional development.

C. The individual shall function within the parameters of his or her competence and the standards of the profession.

D. The individual shall refer clients to other service providers or consult with service providers when additional knowledge and expertise is required.

**Principle 3
(Compliance with
Laws and Regulations)**

Occupational therapy personnel shall comply with laws and Association policies guiding the profession of occupational therapy.

A. The individual shall be acquainted with applicable local, state, federal, and institutional rules and Association policies and shall function accordingly.

B. The individual shall inform employers, employees, and colleagues about those laws and policies that apply to the profession of occupational therapy.

C. The individual shall require those whom they supervise to adhere to the Code of Ethics.

D. The individual shall accurately record and report information.

**Principle 4
(Public Information)**

Occupational therapy personnel shall provide accurate information concerning occupational therapy services.

A. The individual shall accurately represent his or her competence and training.

B. The individual shall not use or participate in the use of any form of communication that contains a false, fraudulent, deceptive, or unfair statement or claim.

**Principle 5
(Professional
Relationships)**

Occupational therapy personnel shall function with discretion and integrity in relations with colleagues and other professionals, and shall be concerned with the quality of their services.

A. The individual shall report illegal, incompetent, and/or unethical practice to the appropriate authority.

B. The individual shall not disclose privileged information when participating in reviews of peers, programs, or systems.

C. The individual who employs or supervises colleagues shall provide appropriate supervision, as defined in AOTA guidelines or state laws, regulations, and institutional policies.

D. The individual shall recognize the contributions of colleagues when disseminating professional information.

Principle 6 (Professional Conduct) Occupational therapy personnel shall not engage in any form of conduct that constitutes a conflict of interest or that adversely reflects the profession.

C: *Theoretical Foundation*

The theoretical foundation of occupational therapy consists of those theories and empirical data from various disciplines that serve as the theoretical foundation for frames of reference and, thus, for practice. In addition, it includes selected information from the applied body of knowledge of medicine. Although this list is not necessarily complete, the theoretical foundation of the profession is comprised of the following information:

1. From the Biological Sciences
   - Anatomy and physiology
   - Biomechanics and kinesiology
   - Function and dysfunction of the biological systems and change through the life cycle
   - The various relationships between the biological systems
   - Impact of stress on the biological systems
   - The effect of atmospheric elements (light, color, sound, etc.) and the application of heat and cold on biological function

2. From Psychology
   - Characteristics and functions of sensory, perceptual, and cognitive processes and their change over the life cycle
   - Learning and factors influencing learning
   - Psychological needs and the effects of need deprivation
   - Psychosocial, psychosexual, personality, and moral development

- Psychoanalytic theory, ego psychology, and symbolism
- The psychological aspects of the various life stages
- Nature and influence of the nonhuman environment, including atmospheric elements, on psychological function
- The psychological components of disability, acute and chronic illness, dying, death, and loss
- The nature and significance of play and recreation
- Industrial psychology
- Psychological aspects of stress

3. From Sociology
- Communication
- Dynamics of one-to-one interactions
- Structure and process of primary groups and how such groups can be directed towards facilitating growth, satisfying needs, and maintaining function
- The nature of secondary groups and larger social systems
- Socialization process and deviance
- The nature and function of social roles
- Dynamics of family and friend relationships
- The nature of work
- Occupational choice, patterns of career development and change, and retirement
- Cultural and social similarities and differences in life styles, values, and norms

4. From Medicine
- The sequelae of genetic deficit, disease, trauma, and stress
- Aspects of medical treatment, course, and prognoses of those diagnostic categories of concern to occupational therapists that are likely to influence intervention
- The therapeutic and nontherapeutic effects of common medications

D: Domain of Concern

T he domain of concern of occupational therapy is comprised of various social roles and the skills that permit and support participation in these roles. The following taxonomy is only an outline of the profession's domain of concern and is not intended to be an all-inclusive or definitive statement about the profession's areas of expertise.

There are three major categories within this taxonomy. The first two—occupational performance areas and performance components—are those aspects of human experience toward which intervention is directed. Performance components are the building blocks of occupational performance areas. Once the components are mastered, they are integrated, elaborated, refined, combined, and recombined in a variety of ways that enable the individual to engage in the multiple activities inherent in the various occupational performance areas. For example, one performance component, "initiating, sustaining, and terminating activities," may be used alone and/or combined with other components, such as "dyadic interaction," in participating in aspects of occupational performance areas like "personal hygiene" and "completion of assigned work."

However, the activities inherent in occupational performance areas are more than the sum of their performance components. Many of these activities, because of their complexity or uniqueness or because of a client's particular problems, must be directly learned—for example, how to go about seeking and acquiring employment. Therefore, occupational therapy intervention is directed towards both mastery of performance components and occupational performance areas, depending on the needs of a client.

The third major category of the taxonomy—"context"— provides the perspective from which performance components and occupational performance areas are viewed relative to the individual. To a great extent, the elements included in this category—age and environment—are used in part to determine whether an individual is in a state of function or dysfunction and whether intervention is necessary or feasible, and to plan and implement appropriate intervention.

I. Occupational Performance Areas

Areas of occupational performances, sometimes referred to as social roles, are organized patterns of behavior that are characteristic and expected of an individual in a given position within a social system. They are:

A. Family Interaction: Includes those roles such as sibling, aunt, and stepfather that are typically a part of nuclear, extended, and expanded families. Family interaction also includes intimate relationships that are seen by their participants as family-like in nature. This area is concerned with:

1. Age and culturally appropriate behaviors relative to successful interaction in required and/or desired familial roles.

2. Dealing with the familial issues of, and activities related to:

   a. Intimacy.
   b. Emotional support.
   c. Sexuality.
   d. Financial matters.
   e. Child rearing.
   f. Care of family members.

3. Preparation for new familial roles through such interactions as courtship and family planning.

4. Preparation for, and accommodation to, marked changes in a familial role.

B. Activities of Daily Living: Includes those tasks

that must be accomplished in order to participate comfortably in the other occupational performance areas—family interaction, recreation,
and work, for example. These tasks are primary aspects of the roles of caretaker of the self
and of home manager—one who takes responsibility for many of the activities of daily living
of others living in a home:

1. Personal hygiene, grooming, and dressing.
2. Eating.
3. Meal preparation and clean-up.
4. Mobility and travel.
5. Money management.
6. Shopping.
7. Care of clothing.
8. Health care.
9. Home maintenance and safety.
10. Communication necessary for accomplish-
    ing activities of daily living.
11. Locating and using community resources.
12. Selecting and supervising caregivers.

C. Play, Leisure, Recreation, and Friendships:
   Shared or solitary interactions engaged in for
   the purpose of amusement, relaxation, or self-
   actualization. Friendships are included in this
   category because they are an integral part of
   many play, leisure, and recreational activities.

1. Play—This area includes age-appropriate
   activities such as:
   a. Exploratory and movement play.
   b. Imitative play.
   c. Fantasy and make-believe.
   d. Construction activities and art work.
   e. Games.
2. Leisure—Time free from the responsibilities of family interaction, activities of daily
   living, and school/work. Leisure time is
   use for such activities as:
   a. Volunteer work.
   b. Political activities.

    c. Care of spiritual needs.

    d. Rest.

    e. Recreation.

3. Recreation:

    a. Participating in a variety of activities that are of interest to the individual and that are experienced as need-satisfying.

    b. Maintaining a comfortable balance between active and sedentary activities, and between time spent alone and with others.

4. Friendships:

    a. Forming friend relationships.

    b. Regular involvement with a variety of people who are described as friends.

    c. Friend relationships that vary on a continuum from casual to close.

D. School and Work: This area includes the various interactions involved in being a student and participating in remunerative employment:

1. School

    a. Class attendance.

    b. Classroom interactions.

    c. Relationships with teachers, classmates, and administrators.

    d. Preparation for classes.

    e. Academic performance.

2. Work

    a. Awareness of personal assets, limitations, likes and dislikes relative to work.

    b. Age-appropriate activities relative to making an appropriate occupational choice.

    c. Seeking and acquiring employment.

    d. Work habits: Attendance, punctuality, relationship with coworkers and supervisors, completion of assigned work, compliance with the norms of the work setting.

e. Management of bureaucratic structures.

f. Preparation for, and adjustment to, retirement.

II. Performance Components

Performance components are basic skills that enable the individual to participate in the various occupational performance areas. They are the building blocks for occupational performances:

A. Biological Components: Those sensory, motor, perceptual and physiological processes that are fundamental to engaging in functional activities.

1. Sensory Integration—Processing of information from the tactile, proprioceptive, vestibular, visual, auditory, gustatory, and olfactory sensory systems.

2. Perception—Stereognosis, kinesthesia, right-left discrimination, form consistency, position in space, visual closure, figure-ground recognition, depth perception, and topographical orientation.

3. Neuromuscular Processes—Reflexes, muscle tone, postural control, laterality, bilateral integration, praxis, gross and fine motor coordination, visual motor integration, and oral motor control.

4. Motor Processes—Range of motion, strength, endurance, and activity tolerance.

5. Soft Tissue Integration—Anatomical and physiological conditions of interstitial tissue and skin.

B. Cognitive Components: The ability to use information for the purpose of thinking, planning, and problem solving:

1. Alertness, orientation, memory, and concentration.

2. Sequencing, categorizing, concept formation, and mathematical calculation.

3. Initiating, sustaining, and terminating activities.

4. Synthesis, generalization, and transfer of learning.

5. Problem solving and planning.

6. Time management.

7. An age-appropriate fund of general information.

C. Psychological Components:The ability to reach and maintain a comfortable level of emotional equilibrium; to monitor one's behavior; and to view oneself, others, and one's life situation realistically:

1. Appropriate expression of needs, values, emotions, and interests.

2. Dealing with adverse experiences such as success/failure, frustration, anxiety, anger, loss, and mourning.

3. Self-discipline—includes volition, self-control, responsibility for self, and self-direction.

4. Appropriate defense mechanisms, reality testing, and insight.

5. Self-concept—an umbrella term that includes identity, sexual identity, body image, knowledge of one's assets and limitations, and self-esteem.

6. Concept of others—ideas and feelings about people in general, particular classes or types of people, and specific people significant to the self.

D. Social Components: Those abilities that allow one to engage with others in casual and sustained relationships, individually and within the context of a variety of small groups.

1. Interpretation of situations—astute observation of social situations, including the feelings of others, and of the behavioral expectations of social situations.

2. Social skills—includes verbal and nonverbal communication, dyadic interaction, and group interaction.

3. Structured social interplay—engaging in situations that require cooperation, competition, negotiation, compromise, and assertiveness.

III. Context

A. Age: Refers to periods of human life measured by years from birth and/or by activities:

   1. Chronological—Age of the individual relative to the date of conception or birth.

   2. Developmental—An individual's capacity to function in specific areas relative to formal or informal norms of his or her cultural group.

   3. Place in the life cycle—An individual's involvement in one or more major life events that are not closely related to chronological age, such as giving birth, making a career change, or starting graduate school.

B. Environment: Refers to people, things, events, and ideas that directly or indirectly affect an individual:

   1. Cultural—A cultural system consists of the social structures, beliefs, values, standards of behavior, customs, and expectations that are accepted and shared by a group of people. An individual is influenced by past, present, and expected future involvement in various cultural systems.

   2. Social—The matrix of people with whom an individual is presently involved or will be involved with in the future, including family, friends, neighbors, coworkers, and individuals who provide care and services.

   3. Physical—The nonhuman environment in which an individual exists or will exist, including food, clothing, technological products, and shelter; possible architectural barriers; the complexity of the environment; degree of physical safety; and nonhuman objects that have personal meaning to the individual, such as dolls, family pictures, or books.

To gain a somewhat different perspective regarding occupational therapy's domain of concern, the reader may wish to examine the *Uniform Terminology for Occupational Therapy—Second Edition* (American Occupational Therapy Association, 1989)—hereafter referred to as Uniform Terminology/2—and its application to practice as described by Dunn and McGourty (1989). Although not labelled as such, the Uniform Terminology/2 does seem to be a delineation of the profession's domain of concern.

Although many similarities exist between the above-outlined taxonomy and Uniform Terminology/2, there are three noteworthy differences. First, Uniform Terminology/2 does not include "Family Interaction" as one of the occupational performance area categories. This is probably due to the strong tradition of the ADL-work-play/leisure triad, rather than an attempt to exclude occupational therapists from assisting clients in family interaction.

Second, in Uniform Terminology/2, performance components are described as being the focus of intervention, to the exclusion of occupational performance areas. Occupational performance areas seem to be viewed primarily as the boundaries of the profession's domain of concern rather than as of direct concern in intervention. The domain of concern appears to be limited to deficits in performance components that interfere with participation in one or more of the specified occupational performance areas. Moreover, problems in occupational performance areas that are not grounded in performance component deficit are not described as part of the profession's domain of concern. Third, Uniform Terminology/2 does not include the categories of "Age" and "Environment." This is probably due more to the universal acceptance of these areas as being fundamental to occupational therapy's domain of concern, evaluation, and interventions than to any implication of their lack of importance.

Finally, as described in Chapter 8, it is very difficult to formulate a taxonomy without flaws. This is particularly true in the case of occupational therapy's domain of concern because of its breadth, complexity, and multidimensional quality.

Ideally, a profession's domain of concern clearly identifies and labels problems of concern to the profession. It is stated so as to reflect the profession's current sets of guidelines for practice and areas having potential for serving as the nucleus for new sets of guidelines for practice. Conversely, the statement of a domain of concern should not be so highly structured that enigmatic problems cannot be identified or reconceptualized from a different perspective. It is difficult and rare to arrive at this ideal state.

E: Legitimate Tools

The legitimate tools of occupational therapy are those activities, actions, instruments, modalities, methods, and processes in which members of the profession have expertise, and which they use as the media for assisting clients.[1]

Legitimate tools are used as a means to accomplish some end. They should not be confused with the goals of intervention, such as grooming activities engaged in for the express purpose of mastering various aspects of grooming. In this sense, grooming is a skill to be learned, not a means for reaching some different end. Grooming would be considered a tool if it were used as the medium for assisting in remediating cognitive deficits. Moreover, legitimate tools should not be confused with specific techniques derived from a particular frame of reference, such as strengthening

---

[1] Two aspects of occupational therapy previously included by the author in the list of legitimate tools—"the teaching-learning process" and "activity analysis and synthesis"—are not included here. The teaching-learning process is part of many frames of reference in occupational therapy. The theoretical information that supports this process—learning theories—is more appropriately placed in the theoretical foundation of the profession. Activity analysis and synthesis, grounded in the profession's frames of reference, are a series of intellectual processes facilitating selection of appropriate tools for problem identification and resolution with clients. Thus, it is more appropriately placed in "practice," the third level of the profession's fundamental body of knowledge.

exercises, or with an entire frame of reference, such as "Bobath techniques."

Legitimate tools are generic in the sense that they are not related to any specific frame of reference. They are selected and combined in a variety of ways depending on the guidelines outlined in various frames of reference. Although there continues to be considerable controversy regarding what constitutes a legitimate tool of occupational therapy, the following is one way of identifying and categorizing the tools used by the profession at this time:[2]

I. Interpersonal Processes

A. Conscious use-of-self: Listening, questioning, clarifying, giving information, instructing, taking a specific attitude or stance, and so forth.

B. Activity groups: Of various levels of sophistication, involving the use of activities and/or discussion of current or anticipated actions within an occupational performance area.

II. Activity Processes

A. Components of occupational performance areas—Meal preparation/eating, shopping, sports, games, arts and crafts, simulated work activities, and so forth.

B. Stimulus-response activities—Sensory stimulation, handling, positioning, massage, exercise, biofeedback, and so forth.

III. Physical Modalities

A. Atmospheric elements—Space, light, color, temperature, sound, and so forth.

B. Technological products—Prosthetic and orthotic devices; splints; seating systems; self-help devices and gadgets; computer hardware, attachments, and software; and so forth.

C. Physical agents—Heat and cold delivered through various means.

---

[2] Based in part on the work of Esther Yuk-mui Nam, Flora Suet-fong Tsang, and Patton Hing-man Wu. (Summer 1990). Class project, E40.2763. New York University.

References

Ackerknecht, E. H. (1968). *A short history of medicine*. New York: Ronald Press.

Allen, C. (1974). Commentary. In H. J. Steffins & H. N. Muller, III (Eds.), *Science, technology and culture* (pp. 22-24). New York: AMS Press.

Allen, C. K. (1985). *Occupational therapy for psychiatric diseases: Measurement and management*. Boston: Little, Brown.

Altmaier, E. M., & Meyer, M. E. (1985). Introduction. In E. M. Altmaier & M. E. Meyer (Eds.), *Applied specialties in psychology* (pp. 1-15). New York: Random House.

American Occupational Therapy Association. (1988). Occupational therapy code of ethics. *American Journal of Occupational Therapy, 42*, 795-796.

American Occupational Therapy Association. (1989). Uniform terminology for occupational therapy (2nd ed.). *American Journal of Occupational Therapy, 43*, 808-815.

American Psychiatric Association. (1987). *Diagnostic and statistical manual of mental disorders* (3rd ed., rev.). Washington, DC: Author.

Anderson, B., & Bell, J. (1988). *Occupational therapy: Its place in Australia's history*. Melbourne: New South Wales Association of Occupational Therapists.

Argyris, C., & Schon, D. A. (1974). *Theory in practice: Increasing professional effectiveness*. San Francisco: Jossey-Bass.

Ausubel, D. P. (1953). The nature of educational research. *Educational Theory, 3*, 314-320.

Ayres, A. J. (1979). *Sensory integration and the child*. Los Angeles: Western Psychological Services.

Bandura, A. (1977). *Social learning theory*. Englewood Cliffs, NJ: Prentice-Hall.

Beauchamp, T. L., & Childress, J. F. (1983). *Principles of biomedical ethics* (2nd ed.). New York: Oxford University Press.

Beckstrand, J. (1986). The notion of a practice theory and the relationship of scientific and ethical knowledge to practice. In L. H. Nicoll (Ed.), *Perspectives on nursing theory* (pp. 481-488). Boston: Little, Brown.

Bertalanffy, L. von. (1967). *General systems theory*. New York: George Braziller.

Blungart, H. L. (1973). Medicine: The art and science. In R. J. Bulger (Ed.), *Hippocratic revisited* (pp. 3-42). New York: Medcom.

Bobath, B. (1979). *Adult hemiplegia: Evaluation and treatment* (2nd ed.). London: Heinemann Medical Books.

Bouton, K. (1989, January 29). The Nobel pair. *New York Times Magazine*, pp. 27-28, 60, 82, 86-88.

Branscomb, L. M. (1973). Conducting and using research. *Daedalus, 102*(2), 145-152.

Brody, B. A. (1988). *Life and death decision making*. Oxford: Oxford University Press.

Brooks, H. (1988). The research university: Doing good and doing it better. *Issues in Science and Technology, 4*(2), 49-55.

Broudy, H. S., Ennis, H. R., & Krimerman, L. I. (Eds.). (1973). *Philosophy of educational research*. New York: Wiley.

Bucher, R., & Strauss, A. L. (1961). Professions in process. *American Journal of Sociology, 66*, 325-334.

Bunge, M. (1983). Towards a philosophy of technology. In C. Mitcham & R. Mackey (Eds.), *Philosophy and technology: Readings in the philosophical problems of technology* (pp. 62-76). Glencoe, NY: The Free Press.

Burbidge, G. (1992). Essay—Why only one big bang? *Scientific American, 266*(2), 120.

Campbell, A. (1980). Comments by Angus Campbell. In W. K. Frankena (Ed.), *The philosophy and future of graduate education* (pp. 173-175). Ann Arbor: University of Michigan Press.

Capron, A. M. (1989). Human experimentation. In R. M. Veatch (Ed.), *Medical ethics* (pp. 125-172). Boston: Jones and Bartlett.

Carroll, J. B. (1968). Basic and applied research in education: Definitions, distinctions, and implications. *Harvard Education Review, 38,* 263-276.

Cassidy, H. G. (1962). *The science and the arts: A new alliance.* New York: Harper & Brothers.

Childress, J. F. (1989). The normative principles of medical ethics. In R. M. Veatch (Ed.), *Medical ethics* (pp. 27-63). Boston: Jones and Bartlett.

Christiansen, C. H. (1990). Guest editorial: The perils of plurality. *Occupational Therapy Journal of Research, 10,* 259-265.

Collins, R. M., & Fielder, J. H. (1986). Beckstrand's concept of practice theory: A critique. In L. H. Nicoll (Ed.), *Perspectives on nursing theory* (pp. 505-511). Boston: Little John.

Cronbach, L. (1985). Essentials of psychological testing (4th ed.). New York: Harper & Row.

Degler, C. M. (1991). *In search of human nature: The decline and revival of Darwinism in American social thought.* New York: Oxford University Press.

Dickoff, J., & James, P. (1968). A theory of theories: A position paper. *Nursing Research, 17,* 197-203.

Diesing, P. (1982). *Science and ideology in the policy sciences.* New York: Aldine.

Dingwall, R. (1982). Introduction. In R. Dingwall (Ed.), *The sociology of professions: Lawyers, doctors and others* (pp. 1-13). New York: St. Martin's Press.

Dowie, J., & Elstein, A. (1988). Introduction. In J. Dowie & A. Elstein (Eds.), *Professional judgement: A reader in clinical decision making* (pp. 1-41). Cambridge: Cambridge University Press.

Downs, F. S. (1979). Clinical and theoretical research. In F. S. D owns & J. W. Fleming (Eds.), *Issues in nursing research* (pp. 67-87). New York: Appleton-Century-Crofts.

Dunn, W., & McGrourty, L. (1989). Application of uniform technology in practice. *American Journal of Occupational Therapy, 43,* 817-831.

Eddy, D. M., & Clanton, C. H. (1982). The art of diagnosis: Solving the clinicopathological exercise. *New England Journal of Medicine, 306,* 1263-1268.

Edwards, R. B., & Graber, G. C. (1988). Ethical foundations. In R. B. Edwards & G. C. Graber (Eds.), *Bio-ethics* (pp. 1-8). San Diego: Harcourt Brace Jovanovich.

Etzioni, A. (Ed.). (1969). *The semi-professions and their organization: Teachers, nurses and social workers.* Glencoe, NY: The Free Press.

Feibleman, J. K. (1983). Pure science, applied science and technology: An attempt at definition. In C. Mitcham & R. Mackey (Eds.), *Philosophy and technology: Readings in the philosophical problems of technology* (pp. 33-41). Glencoe, NY: The Free Press.

Feynman, R. P. (1985). *"Surely you're joking Mr. Feynman!"* New York: W. W. Norton.

Fitzpatrick, J. J., & Whall, A. L. (1983). Overview of nursing models. In J. J. Fitzpatrick & A. L. Whall (Eds.), *Conceptual models for nursing: Analysis and application* (pp. 1-10). Bowie, MD: Robert J. Brady.

Fleming, M. H., Johnson, J. A., Marina, M., Spergel, E. L., & Townson, B. (1987). *Occupation therapy: Directions for the future.* Rockville, MD: American Occupational Therapy Association.

Flexner, A. (1910). *Medical education in the United States and Canada* (Bulletin No. 4). New York: Carnegie Foundation for the Advancement of Teaching.

Flexner, S. B., & Hauck, L. C. (Eds.). (1987). *The Random House dictionary of the English language* (2nd ed.). New York: Random House.

Foss, L., & Rothenberg, K. (1987). *The second medical revolution.* Boston: New Science Library.

Fox, R. E. (1986). Professional preparation: The gap between education and practice. In H. Dorken & Associates (Eds.), *Professional psychology in transition* (pp. 121-140). San Francisco: Jossey-Bass.

Galdston, I. (1981). *Social and historical foundations for modern medicine.* New York: Brunner/Mazel.

Glaser, R. (1976). Cognitive psychology and instructional design. In D. Klahr (Ed.), *Cognition and instruction* (pp. 303-315). New York: Wiley.

Glazer, M. (1980). The disciplinary and the professional in graduate school education in the social sciences. In W. K. Frankena (Ed.), *The philosophy and future of graduate education* (pp. 160-172). Ann Arbor: University of Michigan Press.

Goldstein, T. (1988). *Dawn of modern science.* Boston: Houghton Mifflin.

Goodlad, S. (1984). Introduction. In S. Goodlad (Ed.), *Education for the professions: Quis custodiet* (pp. 3-16). Worcester, Great Britain: The Society for Research in Higher Education & N FER-NELSON.

Gould, S. J. (1989, July 30). Judging the perils of official hostility to scientific error. *The New York Times (The Week in Review)*, p. 6.

Graber, G. C., & Thomasma, D. C. (1989). *The theory and practice of medical ethics.* New York: Continuum.

Greene, M. (1973). *Teacher as a stranger: Educational philosophy for the modern age.* Belmont, CA: Wadsworth.

Grove, J. W. (1989). *In defence of science: Science, technology, and politics in modern society.* Toronto: University of Toronto Press.

Gurin, A., & Williams, D. (1973). Social work education. In E. C. Hughes, B. Thorns, A. M. DeBaggis, A. Gurin, & D. Williams (Eds.), *Education for the professions of medicine, law, theology and social welfare* (pp. 201-247). New York: McGraw-Hill.

Habermas, J. (1973). *Theory and practice.* Boston: Beacon Press.

Hansen, R. A. (Ed.). (1988). Special issue on ethics [Special issue]. *American Journal of Occupational Therapy, 42*(5).

Hansen, R. A. (1989). Ethical considerations. In C. B. Royeen (Ed.), *AOTA self-study series.* Rockville, MD: American Occupational Therapy Association.

Hardy, M. E. (1973). Nature of theories. In M. E. Hardy (Ed.), *Theoretical foundations for nursing* (pp. 10-22). New York: MSS Information.

Hellemans, A., & Bunch, B. (1988). *The timetables of science.* New York: Simon and Schuster.

Henderson, A. (1988). Occupational therapy knowledge: From practice to theory. 1988 Eleanor

Clarke Slagle lecture. *American Journal of Occupational Therapy, 42,* 567-576.

Hilgard, E. R., & Bower, G. H. (1974). *Theories of learning* (4th ed.). Englewood Cliffs, NJ: Prentice-Hall.

Hilts, P. J. (1991, March 31). The Imanishi-Kari case: Can the scales of justice be calibrated for scientific fraud?. *The New York Times (The Week in Review),* p. 7.

Horgan, J. (1988). Physiology of medicine. *Scientific American, 259*(6), 33.

Hughes, E. C. (1973). Introduction. In E. C. Hughes, B. Thorne, A. M. DeBaggis, A. Gurin, & D. Williams (Eds), *Education for the professions of medicine, law, theology and social welfare* (pp. 1-16). New York: McGraw-Hill.

Hull, R. (1988). Codes or no codes. In R. B. Edwards & G. C. Graber (Eds.), *Bio-ethics,* (pp. 45-50). San Diego: Harcourt Brace Jovanovich.

Ihde, D. (1983). The historical-ontological properties of technology over science. In P. T. Durbin & F. Rapp (Eds.), *Philosophy and technology* (pp. 235-253). Boston: D. Reidel Publishing.

Jarvie, I. C. (1983). The social character of technological problems: Comments on Skolimowski's paper. In C. Mitcham & R. Mackey (Eds.), *Philosophy and technology: Readings in the philosophical problems of technology* (pp. 50-53). Glencoe, NY: The Free Press.

Jarvie, I. C. (1986). *Thinking about society: Theory and practice.* Boston: D. Reidel Publishing.

Kassirer, J. P., Kuipers, B. J., & Gorry, G. A. (1982). Towards a theory of clinical expertise. *American Journal of Medicine, 73,* 251-259.

Kerlinger, F. N. (1960, March 26). The mythology of educational research: The methods approach. *School and Society, 88,* 102-107.

Kerlinger, F. N. (1986). *Foundations of behavioral research* (3rd ed.). New York: Holt, Rinehart & Winston.

Kielhofner, G. (1983). A paradigm for practice: The hierarchical organization of occupational therapy knowledge. In G. Kielhofner (Ed.), *Health through occupation: Theory and practice in occupational therapy* (pp. 55-91). Philadelphia: F. A. Davis.

King, T. (1981). *A theory for nursing: Systems, concepts, process*. New York: Wiley.

Kneller, G. F. (1978). *Science as a human endeavor*. New York: Columbia University Press.

Kuhn, T. (1970). *The structure of scientific revolutions* (2nd ed.). Chicago: University of Chicago Press.

Larsen, J. K. (1981). Knowledge utilization. In R. F. Rich (Ed.), *The knowledge cycle* (pp. 149-167). Beverly Hills: Sage.

Larsen, M. S. (1977). *The rise of professionalism: A sociological analysis*. Berkeley: University of California Press.

Lieb, I. (1986). *Linking theory, research and practice*. In H. K. Grant (Ed.), Occupational therapy education: Target 2000 (pp. 113-118). Rockville, MD: American Occupational Therapy Association.

Llorens, L. A., & Gillette, N. P. (1985). The challenge for research in a practice profession. *American Journal of Occupational Therapy, 39*, 143-145.

Lowe, V. (1962). *Understanding Whitehead*. Baltimore: Johns Hopkins University Press.

Lusted, L. B. (1968). *Introduction to medical decision making*. Springfield, IL: Charles C. Thomas.

McGlothlin, W. (1964). *The professional schools*. New York: Center for Applied Research in Education.

Magraw, R. M. (1973). Science and humanism: Medicine and existential anguish. In R. J. Bulger (Ed.), *Hippocratic revisited* (pp. 43-49). New York: Medcom.

Marx, M. H., & Cronan-Hillix, W. A. (1987). *Systems and theories in psychology* (4th ed.). New York: McGraw-Hill.

Merton, R. K. (1968). *Social theory and social structure*. Glencoe, NY: The Free Press.

Merton, R. K. (1982). *Social research and the practicing professions*. Cambridge, MA: Apt Books.

Mills, C. E. (1967). *The sociological imagination*. New York: Oxford University Press.

Mitcham, C., & Mackey, R. (1983). Introduction: Technology as a philosophical problem. In C. Mitcham & R. Mackey (Eds.), *Philosophy and technology: Readings in the philosophical problems of technology* (pp. 1-30). Glencoe, NY: The Free Press.

Moore, W. E. (1970). *The professions: Roles and rules.* New York: Russell Sage Foundation.

Mosey, A. C. (1981). *Occupational therapy: Configuration of a profession.* New York: Raven Press.

Mosey, A. C. (1985). Eleanor Clarke Slagle lecture, 1985: A monistic or a pluralistic approach to professional identity. *American Journal of Occupational Therapy, 39,* 504-509.

Mosey, A. C. (1986). *Psychosocial components of occupational therapy.* New York: Raven Press.

Mosey, A. C. (1989). Guest editorial. The proper focus of scientific inquiry: Frames of reference. *Occupational Therapy Journal of Research, 9,* 195-201.

Nam, E. Y., Tsang, F. S., & Patton, H. W. (Summer 1990). Class project, E40.2763. New York University.

Newman, M. A. (1986). Nursing's theoretical evolution. In L. H. Nicoll (Ed.), *Perspectives on nursing* (pp. 72-78). Boston: Little John.

Pellegrino, E. D. (1979). The anatomy of clinical judgments. In H. T. Engelhardt, S. F. Specker, & B. Towers (Eds.), *Clinical judgement: A critical appraisal* (pp. 169-194). Boston: D. Reidel Publishing.

Perutz, M. F. (1989). *Is science necessary? Essays on science and scientists.* New York: E. P. Dutton.

Phillips, D. C. (1987). *Philosophy, science, and social inquiry.* Oxford: Pergamon.

Popper, K. (1968). *Conjectures and refutations: The growth of scientific knowledge.* New York: Harper and Row.

Regis, E. (1987). *Who got Einstein's office?* Reading, MA: Addison-Wesley.

Rodgers, D. A. (1986). Psychologists as practitioners, not technicians. In H. Dorken & Associates (Eds.), *Professional psychology in transition* (pp. 141-173). San Francisco: Jossey-Bass.

Rogers, J. C. (1983). Clinical reasoning: The ethics, science and art. *American Journal of Occupational Therapy, 37,* 601-616.

Rogers, M. E. (1970). *An introduction to the theoretical basis of nursing.* Philadelphia: F. A. Davis.

Rollin, B. E. (1988). The use and abuse of animals in research. In R. B. Edwards & G. C. Graber (Eds.), *Bio-ethics* (pp. 231-245). San Diego: Harcourt Brace Jovanovich.

Rood, M. (1954). Neurophysiological reactions as a basis for physical therapy. *Physical Therapy Review, 34*, 444-449.

Rosenberg, C. E. (1976). *No other gods: On science and American social thought.* Baltimore: John Hopkins University Press.

Rosenberg, N., & Birdzell, L. E., Jr. (1990). Science, technology and the western miracle. *Scientific American, 293*(5), 42-54.

Rule, J. B. (1978). *Insight and social betterment: A preface to applied social science.* New York: Oxford University Press.

Schein, E. H. (1972). *Professional education.* New York: McGraw-Hill.

Schon, D. A. (1983). *The reflective practitioner: How professionals think in action.* New York: Basic Books.

Schwartz, D. M. (1989). It takes more than repellent to make flying pests bug off. *Smithsonian, 20*(4), 79-87.

Scott, R. A., & Shore, A. R. (1979). *Why sociology does not apply: A study of the use of sociology in public policy.* New York: Elsevier.

Shapere, D. (1984). *Reason and the search for knowledge: Investigations in the philosophy of science.* Boston: D. Reidel Publishing.

Singleton, R., Jr., Straits, B. C., Straits, M. M., & McAllister, R. J. (1988). *Approaches to social research.* New York: Oxford University Press.

Skolimowski, H. (1983). The structure of thinking in technology. In C. Mitcham & R. Mackey (Eds.), *Philosophy and technology: Readings in the philosophical problems of technology* (pp. 42-49). Glencoe, NY: The Free Press.

Snelbecker, G. E. (1974). *Learning theory, instructional theory and psycho-educational design.* New York: McGraw-Hill.

Tempkin, O. (1977). *The double face of Janus.* Baltimore: John Hopkins University Press.

Thorne, B. (1973). Professional education in medicine. In E. C. Hughes, B. Thorne, A. M. DeBaggis, A. Gurin, & D. Williams (Eds.), *Education for the professions of medicine, law, theology and social welfare* (pp. 17-99). New York: McGraw-Hill.

Van Melsen, A. G. (1961). *Science and technology* (Duquesne Studies, Philosophical Series 13). Pittsburgh: Duquesne University Press.

Veatch, R. M. (1989) Medical ethics: An introduction. In R. M. Veatch (Ed.), *Medical ethics* (pp. 1-26). Boston: Jones and Bartlett.

Vockell, E. L. (1983). *Educational research*. London: MacMillan.

Wartofsky, M. W. (1979). *Models: Representation and scientific understanding*. Boston: D. Reidel Publishing.

Weissman, G. (1991). Aspirin. *Scientific American, 265*(1), 84-90.

Williams, L. P. (1974a). Science vs. scientific technology. In H. J. Steffins & H. N. Muller, III (Eds.), *Science, technology and culture* (pp. 8-21). New York: AMS Press.

Williams, L. P. (1974b). Response. In H. J. Steffins & H. N. Muller, III (Eds.), *Science, technology and culture* (pp. 31-42). New York: AMS Press.

Wollmer, H., & Mills, D. (Eds.). (1966). *Professionalism*. Englewood Cliffs, NJ: Prentice-Hall.

Wulff, H. R., Pedersen, S. A., & Rosenberg, R. (1986). *Philosophy of medicine*. Oxford: Blackwell Scientific Publications.

Yerxa, E. J. (1981). Basic or applied? A "developmental assessment" of occupational therapy research. *American Journal of Occupational Therapy, 35,* 820-821.

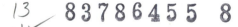